The *navCare* Pocket Guide

Navigating and Communicating in Healthcare & Other Systems

Harry van Bommel

Volume 1 in the 7-Volume
navCare Series

All of the *navCare* materials are dedicated to the members, clients, caregivers, professionals, staff and volunteers of the collaborative partners. What we have learned together is now being shared with anyone who wishes to benefit.

In memory of **Peter Dill** whose unexpected death in 2014 year saddened us all. He was a founding partner of the *navCare* collaborative project and the Executive Director of the Durham Association of Family Respite Services at the time of his death. Most importantly we will remember him for his high principles represented in our working philosophy, his questions that always brought us back to how our work can benefit everyone involved and his genuine, personal attention to the suffering and joys we all experience. Peter was a systems navigator who never forgot that relationship building is an integral part of this role.

The *navCare* Pocket Guide

Navigating and Communicating in Healthcare & Other Systems

One at a Time Press
Oshawa 2015

A Collaborative Project of:

ALS Canada
Better Living Health and Community Services
Caregiver Omnimedia Inc.
Deohaeko Support Network
Durham Association for Family Respite Services
Durham Family Network
Hospice Toronto
Metropolitan United Church
Parkinson Society Central & Northern Ontario
Patients Canada
Saint Elizabeth Health Care
Sykes Assistance Services Corp

We are a consensus-based, inter-professional, and community representative group.

NavCare: www.navCare.org

Some of the materials for this pocket guide are adapted from *Practical Leadership* and *Caring for Loved Ones at Home* with permission of the author, Harry van Bommel of PSD Consultants in Toronto: www.carelibrary.com.

Cover mosaic by Tim van Horn at www.canadianmosaic.ca

Library and Archives Canada
Cataloguing in Publication
van Bommel, Harry, author
NavCare.
Reprint. Originally published: Toronto, Canada : PSD Consultants, 2014.
Includes bibliographical references and indexes.
Contents: Volume 1. The navCare pocket guide : navigating and communicating in health care & other systems / Harry van Bommel -- Volume 2. The navCare textbook : systems navigation, negotiation, and mediation / Harry van Bommel – Volume 3. The navCare hospital and homecare notebook / Harry van Bommel and Janet Klees -- Volume 4. The navCare developing a comprehensive personal profile / Janet Klees -- Volume 5. The navCare personal and family information binder / Harry van Bommel -- Volume 6. The navCare systems information binder / Harry van Bommel -- Volume 7. The navCare templates binder / Harry van Bommel.

**ISBN 978-0-9947412-0-2 (paperback : v. 1).--ISBN 978-0-9947412-1-9 (paperback : v. 2).--
ISBN 978-0-9947412-2-6 (paperback : v. 3).--ISBN 978-0-9947412-3-3 (paperback : v. 4).--
ISBN 978-0-9947412-4-0 (paperback : v. 5).--ISBN 978-0-9947412-5-7 (paperback : v. 6).--
ISBN 978-0-9947412-6-4 (paperback : v. 7).--ISBN 978-0-9947412-7-1 (paperback : set)**

1. Medical care--Canada--Handbooks, manuals, etc. I. Klees, Janet, 1959-, author II. navCare, issuing body III. Title.

RA395.C3V35 2015
362.10971 C2015-902859-0

This information is a service provided by *navCare: a collaborative project by the members listed on the title page*. This material provides information under a Creative Common license. Like any printed material, it may become out of date over time. This information is not intended to be a substitute for the advice of healthcare professionals, lawyers, accountants or other professionals in their respective fields.

For further information:

navcare.org@gmail.com

We gratefully acknowledge the very generous financial support of:

Ontario Trillium Foundation

Fondation Trillium de l'Ontario

An agency of the Government of Ontario.
Relève du gouvernement de l'Ontario.

and the following Foundations and Corporations

HABITAT HEALING

The Healing Cycle FOUNDATION

PSD Consultants

SOLO TRAVELER

We also acknowledge the encouragement of:

Rachel Kampus, A/Assistant Deputy Minister, Health System Accountability and Performance Division Ministry of Health and Long-Term Care

Michael J. Aherne, B.Comm, M.Ed., CMC, Co-Founder, Canadian Pallium Project, University of Alberta

Sonja Davie, former President, Children's Aid Society of Peel Region; Former President, United Way of Peel Region; Former President, Hospice of Peel; Former Principal, Davie & Associates (Adult Education Consulting)

George Paul Dienesch, Secretary and Researcher, The Parliamentary Committee on Palliative and Compassionate Care Report *Not to Be Forgotten: Care of Vulnerable Canadians*

Rick Firth, Executive Director, Hospice Palliative Care Ontario

Bill Morris, Executive Director, Ontario 211 Services Corporation

Charmaine C. Williams, Associate Dean Academic and Associate Professor, Factor-Inwentash Faculty of Social Work, University of Toronto

as well as many front-line professionals, volunteers, family caregivers and individuals receiving support services who have encouraged our efforts since our founding in April, 2008.

The *navCare* Series

The *navCare* Series is designed to help people navigate various service systems, negotiate the best care and services possible and mediate problems as they arise. This pocket guide is volume 1 of this series. You may find that this book is all you need. However, you can download all the publications below for free, now or in the future.

1. **The *navCare* Pocket Guide** [Audience: patients, family caregivers]
2. **The *navCare* Textbook** [Audience: advisors, professionals, volunteers, patients, family caregivers]
   Core training resource materials for people who want to learn more in-depth navigation, negotiation and mediation skills. Can be used for staff and volunteer training, college or university courses.
3. **The *navCare* Hospital and Homecare Notebook** [Audience: family caregivers, advisors]
   Notebook to keep track of hospital visits as well as discharge planning and homecare services.

4. **The *navCare* Developing a Comprehensive Personal Profile** [Audience: family caregivers, advisors professionals, volunteers]
   To help family caregivers and advisors provide specific and practical information on how to best support a person at risk.
5. **The *navCare* Personal and Family Information Binder** [Audience: patients and family caregivers]
   Binder to keep all your personal and family information up to date.
6. **The *navCare* Systems Information Binder** [Audience: patients, family caregivers, advisors, professionals, volunteers]
   Personal file system to keep track of information collected on the various systems.
7. **The *navCare* Templates Binder** [advisors, professionals, volunteers]
   Aid to help organizations customize the *navCare* Series for their own use.

Website: *www.navCare.org*

The above books can be freely downloaded. Organizations can revise and translate the books as they like and are encouraged to freely share their revisions. For further information: *navcare.org@gmail.com*.

Table of Contents

Preface

navCare is about ensuring that the excellent care and services available to some people in our communities is available to all. We have been part of this project since 2008 providing our own expertise as well as editing the 7-book series.

The series is generic in that it fits the broadest audience possible. Over time we will be editing the materials more specifically for our own clientele at DAFRS. In the interim, we hope that you customize the materials for your own uses and share what works best for you and your family with us.

The *navCare* motto is *nurture relationships above all else.* This is true in many aspects of our life. When navigating any system it helps to either know someone who works in that system who can help us or to nurture new relationships with people we are just meeting.

The most successful way to navigate systems is through asking the people you know to help. At DAFRS we are building a list of contacts in our communities who have proven most helpful to our clientele. You can help add to the list by letting us know of doctors, lawyers, accountants, nurses, educators, programs and other people that you have found most helpful.

John Ralston Saul wrote: "There is no idea of society more ancient than a circle of friends and there is nothing more predictable than the discovery that the one in need is somehow helping others." Whenever we go through difficult times, it is our circle of friends that will help us through the navigation, negotiation, and mediation processes ahead.

If you have suggestions for how to make these materials even more useful, please write to us at DAFRS (info@dafrs.com) so that we can incorporate your ideas into the next edition of our *navCare* Series.

Best wishes,

Janet Klees
Executive Director
Durham Association for Family Respite Services

Language

The *navCare* material tries to reach a very broad audience of readers including patients/clients, caregivers (family and friends), professionals, volunteers, and the broader community.

We have used "you" to speak directly to the person who uses a healthcare, community, or social service, or a legal aid clinic or financial service.

Advisor can also be a family caregiver, a volunteer from a community agency or within a system, and it can be a professional within a system or hired directly by a person receiving care and support (or their family on their behalf). This person can advise and guide a person with their family caregivers through an individual system or multiple systems.

The central person refers to you, the client, who is receiving care and support.

Family refers to both people who are part of your immediate family and those you define as members of your family through friendship.

Family Caregiver is a term typically used only in health care yet these family members or dear friends support you through all the various systems in which you may be involved. This name may well change over time, but for now, it best represents the person helping someone navigate, negotiate, and mediate your way through various systems.

A ***Navigator*** can be the person receiving care and services and navigates systems on their own behalf. A navigator can also be a family caregiver, a volunteer from a community agency or within a system, and it can be a professional within a system or hired directly by a person receiving care and supports (or their family on their behalf).

Professional refers to all paid providers with a professional degree or qualification. ***Staff*** refers to paid support people such as administrative assistants, front-line support workers, and call center customer service representatives.

Large ***systems*** include healthcare, community and social services, education, finance, governments and legal systems. They are different from a specific institution or service. For example, a family doctor, a hospital, home care, an x-ray clinic, and a long-term care facility are all part of the healthcare system.

Volunteer refers to unpaid individuals who provide services in some form and are supervised by an agency or program.

Introduction

navCare started in 2008 when a group of people from various organizations got together to see if we could figure out how to help people better navigate systems, negotiate the best care and supports together, and mediate problems as they arise.

Our motto is:

Nurture relationships above all else.

Once you have read and practiced some of what we present here, you will see that it all boils down to one concept: nurturing relationships within families and with friends, with professionals, staff, and volunteers, and with anyone who can be helpful and supportive, now and in the future. In return, you offer them the same level of support when they need you.

Many of us in *navCare* have received excellent care and services over the years and now find that we are able to return the favor to some of our former care providers who are looking for information or referrals themselves.

Whether we return the favor to the same person or to someone else in need, our philosophy remains one of mutual care and support.

When we started this project as volunteers in 2008, we started with a core belief:

"Some people get excellent care and services. Everyone should."

This belief leads us to a realistic benchmark for services for all people in need everywhere. If the service is available to some, that service should be the level of excellence we want to give everyone.

Our starting point, then, is identifying what already exists and trying to move as many people to that benchmark as possible.

navCare is about helping individual people going through a specific situation right now. It is not an advocacy group for changing systems – there are other, highly capable organizations doing that already, including some of our *navCare* partners. Our project seeks to help individuals regardless of what system they find themselves in at any time.

There are, at this time, few resources available through online bookstores or public libraries on navigating systems. This work is original and we hope it will influence the development of similar resources, adapted and revised to meet the reader's needs or those of organizations representing a specific audience of readers.

The information in this program is NOT specific to a disease, a legal issue, or a need within the community. It does NOT replicate information already easily available. The material will lead you to the best approaches to get updated information that already exists.

navCare will be the source for how to:

- navigate the various systems in Ontario while providing templates for other regions, provinces and nationalities to adapt for their own needs.
- negotiate the best care and services possible in any circumstance to meet a person's physical, emotional, spiritual, and information needs, as well as those of their families.
- mediate problems that typically arise.

Through thinking about situations, talking with family, friends and colleagues, through planning and practice the following skills will become natural. They will be added to the knowledge and skills you already have.

First Things First

This pocket guide is short but still too long to use quickly. If you need to navigate any system (e.g., healthcare, legal, education, financial) immediately, here are a few quick tips. The rest of the guide will help you do a more thorough job.

Let us presume you need help within the healthcare system. In an emergency, obviously, you will call **911**. If you have more time, call **Telehealth – 1.866.797.0000** – an Ontario government helpline with Registered Nurses taking your calls to help you determine what you should do next. Depending on their advice you would either:

1. go to the nearest hospital emergency department by ambulance or with a family member or friend.

2. see your family doctor within 24-48 hours.
3. go to a neighborhood walk-in medical clinic (Telehealth can tell you where the nearest one is).
4. rest at home and call Telehealth back within 24-48 hours.

Once the immediate concern is taken care of, you can start looking at the rest of this pocket guide for further helpful information about how to choose a medical specialist, how to find which hospital may be best for you, how to get supports in the community for your family if you need them, how to access homecare services, and so much more.

If it is a legal matter at a courthouse that comes up unexpectedly, immediately seek out the duty counsel who can help you navigate next steps.

In education, the first step is to contact the teacher/professor who can direct you to the appropriate person to help with an unexpected event.

It is similar for other systems – go first to a receptionist or front-line staff to ask for their guidance in unexpected events. Follow their leads. If the matter is not resolved to your satisfaction, take the time when you can to do a bit more research on your own.

In all of these cases, take notes. You will see blank note pages at the back of this pocket guide for this purpose. It is easier to write things down at the time they are happening than it is to try to remember them later.

The Natural Authority of Families[1]

Navigating systems can feel quite intimidating at first. Even walking into a large bank or insurance company, a hospital, a courthouse, or a university can feel frightening. Michael Kendrick has written a short article to help families understand the power a

---

[1] Reprinted with permission by Michael Kendrick, Ph.D., an internationally known author and educator in the fields of leadership, quality services, advocacy, safeguards for vulnerable people, and the promotion of community living for people with a disability. [www.kendrickconsulting.org] Kendrick's encouragement to families was published in CRUCIAL TIMES, June 2013 Issue 45, p 12 by Community Resource Unit, Inc., in South Brisbane, Australia (www.cru.org.au). His intent is to highlight the inherent, natural authority that families have in caring for and advocating on behalf of their loved ones.

family's support role. What families can do for their loved ones is unique – no professional can replace the natural authority of families.

- - - - - - - - - -

Consumers of services and their families will find themselves having to work with professionals, bureaucrats, and others in roles of authority. Not uncommonly, the authority of these persons tends to overshadow the authority of "small people." It can sometimes help to remember that families have a natural authority of their own which can go a long way to reducing this power imbalance. In order for this to happen, however, families need to appreciate this natural authority and be willing to act on it. What follows is a brief description of some of the common sources of authority that families can call on when they are acting in the interests of a family member.

The public generally recognizes the **primacy of families** in terms of their responsibility for a person's well-being. In this way, families have the authority to be highly engaged because they also tend to have greater responsibility for the well-being of their family members.

Families have authority (normally) that arises from long-term observation, insight, and personal relationship. They have known their family member the most fully and over the longest period of time. .

Families typically care about or love their relative more than would be true of others, however committed the others may be. Not only do families usually care more but they are also expected to care more.

Families have a stake in outcomes. For example, they have to live with the long-term consequences of service failures to a greater extent than any other party, except, of course, the person themselves.

Families are expected to advocate for their own members. Generally, they are granted considerable presence in the decision-making processes affecting their family members, even where legal formalities do not require it.

The family is an authoritative witness to the performance of professionals and systems and may have special (though not necessarily exclusive) insight into events that take place.

Family members bring to their role **a wide range of talents and experiences** that can give them additional authority on many matters. For example, a parent might also be an expert educator.

Families are often best positioned to **see how everything, in its entirety, adds up in a person's life**. For this reason they can often see the incongruences of different interventions.

Family members are often **free of the vested interests** that call into question the credibility of other parties. Frequently family members are granted a degree of independence that highlights their credibility and purity of motive.

While these common sources of authority do not, in the end, resolve the question of ultimate authority, they do offer families some measure of security that their views should matter as much as, or more than, others who also claim authority in deciding what will happen to a person. Because it is very difficult for a person to advocate if they hold some doubt about the legitimacy of their role, these points may help to strengthen the resolve to persevere and advocate for your family member.

Navigation

Starting Points

Navigation as a process is based on several assumptions:

- We should not have to create a navigation project or train people in navigation. This is being done because systems are typically not user-friendly enough for people to feel comfortable or confident that they will get the services they need at the same level as some valued clients of the service.
- No navigation training process can ensure that clients and their families will get what they want or need, when they need it, in the way they need it, where they need it, at the right cost, and for the right reasons. The best we can hope for by training ourselves and each other is a better chance of getting these things.

- We are at the starting point of this process. There are no other detailed materials online, in bookstores, or in libraries that provide this information. That means we are, at best, able to begin to collect the strategies, knowledge, and skills of how better to navigate systems.

Finding Your Way

Systems navigation is like the paved walking paths on a newly designed lawn between office buildings and the street. For a time, people use the paved paths to get from one building to either the street or another building.

After a time, however, a few people take a shortcut across the lawn. Over time, more and more people start taking the shortcut until well-worn new paths are created.

Regardless of "*Do not walk on the grass*" signs, people inevitably continue to take the shortcuts until a wise landscape architect converts the shortcuts into paved paths and replaces the original paths with grass.

navCare will help people navigate through systems, finding or creating shortcuts until one day systems will incorporate our routes into their designs.

Relationships are almost always better than techniques. The broader your network of family, friends, and contacts, the more likely you will get the services you need.

Navigation in its simplest form is getting from the front door to the right department. In systems, it means finding out the best way to access the services within a large system and, once at the right physical location, negotiating the best services possible.

If it were simple, however, people would not get so frustrated. Often, to get to the right person at the right time and in the right place you need to go from Point A to B to C to D until you get everything right. You will play telephone tag or have electronic communications misplaced or not answered or be shuffled from one person to the next.

We begin this chapter with two important aspects of navigation: the person doing the navigation and the systems involved. Then we will look at a process used by most successful navigators.

First, the person doing the navigating needs to have some specific characteristics in order to be successful.

The Navigator/Advisor

This navigator can be you, one of your family caregivers, a person hired by you (Advisor) or your family, a volunteer from a community agency or institution, or a person within a specific system whose job it is to help people navigate that system.

To help you decide whether you want to navigate on your own or get the support of someone else, here is a list of characteristics of successful navigators. Note that even successful navigators (e.g., nurses or hospital social workers) who are ill may rely on someone to do the navigating for them so they can focus on their health.

Successful navigators/advisors:

- collect and protect a person's whole story rather than just recording specific needs or problems. They do this for the central person, their family, and their care providers so no one loses touch with who the person is individually and within their communities.
- understand what a person wants, needs, and does not want, and helps develop alternative plans according to ever-changing and unpredictable situations including family dynamics, services available

in their geographic region, their finances, and other supports.

- are detail-oriented and keep notes on successful navigation, negotiation, and mediation strategies with specific people and institutions / systems.
- are persistent, understanding that "no" may be either a firm "no" or an opportunity to investigate deeper into getting to a "yes."
- have excellent personal navigation, negotiation, and mediation skills.
- are naturally curious and good at research or know how to get help to research what they need to know.

Later, we will look at how navigators can improve their knowledge and skills. For now, we have established the basics of who this person can be in your life if it is not you.

Once you have a navigator on your side (or you become the navigator yourself), you will need to understand systems.

System Definition and Power Structures

Systems can be relatively large or very large. They are different from organizations. For example, there are many different kinds of care within health care: e.g., acute care, chronic care, a family doctor's care, and palliative care. These kinds of care are done in hospitals, home care, nursing homes and clinics. All of these kinds of care and places of care (organizations), plus the governments and insurance companies that fund it, make up the healthcare systems.

Systems come with three traditional power structures. You need to know the differences because sometimes you have to talk to someone higher up the power structure than the person you are dealing with to get what you need.

The most common power structure is a top-down hierarchy where everyone reports to a supervisor or manager until you get to the top person – typically the CEO (Chief Executive Officer).

In some organizations the titles will be different. The CEO may be called President and everyone at the second level is a Vice-President. In some charitable organizations, the top person is the Executive Director and underneath that position are Directors or Managers of specific functions or programs.

Each of these bureaucracies has a Board of Directors (corporate, non-profit, and charities) that are responsible for deciding on the mission, values, goals, and objectives of an organization. The staff (Presidents/CEOs/Executive Directors, their managers and staff) are responsible for implementing whatever policies or initiatives the Board approves. Often the executive paid people influence the elected boards more than the other way around. However, that may not be true in all organizations.

The second most common power structure is government where the public service leaders report to politicians for their approval of programs and budgets. The structure is similar to the above, except the titles are different and rather than reporting to a Board, bureaucrats report to a municipal council or a provincial/territorial/federal legislature that changes its composition every 3-5 years following an election. Politicians often lead changes but also follow voter trends if they wish to stay in office. This is not as true in power structures in a top-down hierarchy.

The last large power structure is a double-power structure within one system. This is only seen in higher education systems (e.g., universities) and health care. In both, professors or doctors report to a separate power authority from everyone else in the system. In universities, for example, the professors report to their own governing body within the university. All other staff report up the ranks to the university president.

In hospitals, the physicians report to the Chief of Staff. Everyone else including nurses, allied professionals (e.g., occupational and physiotherapists, social workers, chaplains), administration staff, and building maintenance workers reports to the hospital's CEO.

This double power structure can lead to obvious disagreements about who is responsible to whom for patient or student issues. There is a greater "us versus them" mentality than there might be between departments in a single power structure where everyone shares the same ultimate boss.

One of a navigator's key skills is to understand the power structure within whatever system they are navigating. This will allow them to find the shortest path to the right person who can make the right decisions at the right time, in the right way, in the right place, and for the right reasons.

To understand systems, you need to know that each of us will, at one time or another, be involved in almost all of the systems listed below. Just looking at the list can be overwhelming which is why the frustration with not knowing what to do or how to do it can be so great.

Like all journeys, each navigation starts with a first step. For us, that means understanding the systems we are involved in at the moment.

For healthcare purposes, family doctors do not talk very much with specialists and specialists typically do not talk very much with each other. A patient may have six doctors, none of whom are speaking with the others.

Only you, your family, and outside advisors have the whole picture.

If you are involved in trying to get a benefit from a Human Resources Department at work, or an insurance company, or the government, you will likely have to speak to several people in various departments, most of whom do not talk with each other. You may get different answers from each person and you may need to be the person to get those folks to resolve the situation together to your satisfaction.

If you need services from several systems, you will likely be working with people who do not know very much about the other systems and how they can work together. In fact, they may be trained to refer you to the other system to avoid having to provide you the service themselves. You will get a lot of "That's not our fault, Madame. It is the other service's fault. Call them." When you do call the other service, of course, they may blame the first one or a completely different one.

This is where system navigation, negotiation, and mediation come in. You create your own system to meet your needs. You become the core around which all systems revolve. Almost always, you will need someone, or several people, to help you navigate, negotiate, and mediate. These family members, friends, or advisors become the coordinator(s) of care for all services.

Following are the major categories of systems that each and every one of us will access at some point in our lives. Many of these systems are part of our daily lives through our banks, schools, workplaces, government services (e.g., garbage pickup), and, of course, our healthcare systems.

List of Systems

Community and Social Services

- Children's Aid Societies (or child welfare)
- Community programs (including day programs and respite, babysitting, fitness, support groups, nutrition, adult learning, sports)
- Public and Supportive Housing
- Job Support
- Income Support
- Transportation for those without enough money to pay for their own.

Corporate, Employer, Unions, Associations

Each of these may have Human Resource services such as pensions, insurance, disability accommodations, leaves of absence, sick days, and benefits. Some may also have "navigation" services to help you get what you need through, for example, union representatives or veterans' services to modify your home for long-term care needs.

For example, the Canadian Association of Retired Persons (CARP) provides a free healthcare navigation coach to its members. Veterans Affairs covers home renovation costs for their veterans who need a stair lift, wheelchair ramp, or other accommodations.

Customer Service

When things do not go right with a commercial service, you need to get involved with their customer service department. This could be a store or a company that provides you with cable television or internet services, gas and electricity, telephones, or consumer goods.

Education

Elementary, secondary, college, university, private and special training schools are all part of education systems. Within any of these education systems, children may need extra supports when family members are ill or in need. Children also may go through emotional or behavioral difficulties that require extra supports.

Financial

- Banking
- Insurance Programs
- Investments
- Pensions

Governments

- Aboriginal (e.g., self-government, Indian Affairs)
- Federal (e.g., pensions, death benefits)
- Municipal (e.g., public housing, public health)
- Provincial/Territorial/Regional (e.g., developmental services, guardianship, income supplements)
- Ombudsman, Auditor General
- Political (elected officials and their staffs)

Health Care

- Acute Care
- Chronic Care
- Disease/Condition-Specific Organizations & Resources
- Home Care
    - Nursing & Medical
    - Homemaking (house cleaning, cooking, meals)
    - Non-medical personal support: OT (Occupational Therapists), PT (Physiotherapists), RMT (Registered Massage Therapists), PSW (Personal Support Workers), volunteers, and many more.
- Hospice Palliative Care
- Long-term Care
- Mental Health
- Pharmacies
- Rehabilitation
- Support Groups

Legal Services

- Adoption
- Child Custody
- Civil Law Suits
- Criminal
- Divorce
- Small Claims

The best navigation is when you know someone who says, "Don't worry, Bill. We'll arrange everything" - and they do!

That does not happen often. Sometimes, it happens within a system where people know us well and treat us as most of us want to be treated: with respect and timely, high quality service. Still, it does not happen often enough, even in the systems where we work.

The second best navigation is one that is not rushed. If you are in an airplane, you hope that your pilots have planned their navigation to your destination carefully.

For us, the more we plan ahead, the less of a crisis any navigation needs to be. In life and death situations, of course, you call 911 and worry about navigation after getting to the Emergency Department of your hospital.

When it is not an emergency, there are obvious healthcare situations to plan ahead for: birth, childhood healthcare issues, accidents requiring treatment, diseases requiring treatment, recovery and rehabilitation from surgeries or treatments, home care, healthcare issues as we age, hospice palliative care, death and bereavement. Most of us will experience all of these more than once and most of us are still surprised whenever it happens.

In all the other systems, you will likely experience some difficulties with things such as your children's education, insurance claims, small claims court, customer service lineups or telephone wait times, testifying in a legal matter, participating in your local community center, retirement planning or saving for your children's higher education, dealing with a government department for garbage pickup difficulties, road repair, property taxes, and so much more.

We are surrounded by large, impersonal systems. We try to avoid them whenever we can because they are time-consuming and often frustrating. When we need systems, we want them to work efficiently and effectively so we don't have to worry.

Many of us also work in these systems. When we do, we have an opportunity to be a helpful navigator for our clients and customers rather than another cog in the wheel.

We want to concentrate on our lives, not on the large systems that provide us with services – unless we need them. Then we are typically grateful for any positive results we get.

There are, thankfully, many wonderful people within those large systems – you may even be one of them. Finding these people is sometimes a matter of luck and sometimes the result of a referral. *navCare* wants to ensure we find the right people more often than not.

The Navigation Process

We have looked at who can be a navigator if you choose not to do it yourself, the qualities they need to have, and the systems in which they have to work.

Sometimes you simply need to know when a system's offices are open or where they are located. A phone call (many offices have a recorded message instructing you to "press 1 for office hours, press 2 for location") or a website visit will tell you what you need to know – the basics, such as names, addresses, or phone numbers.

The telephone and internet are your best sources for that kind of information.

This pocket guide looks at more complex situations.

Your Perspective

First you need to look at what you want, need, and do not want, and what type of plan you will agree to.

Sometimes family caregivers, in their efforts to help you, may presume they know what you need and, therefore, ignore you. In their hurry to "fix" something or meet a presumed need, they miss what you actually want.

You probably know your needs quite well. It is important that you let your family and friends know what you need and to work with you, as a team, to help you meet those needs.

Dr. Michele Chaban is a renowned social worker in the fields of end-of-life care and mindfulness meditation. Whenever she works with a new client she asks a few basic questions to start the conversation. These open-ended questions may take from fifteen minutes to two hours to answer as each client tells their own story in a different way. As an Advisor, Dr. Chaban wants to get the whole picture rather than just a list of problems or concerns. She understands that often the patient knows these things without being asked. However, not all patients do and sometimes it can help to go through this process with someone else. Other times patients know what they need but have difficulty expressing it to their family and other caregivers.

In Dr. Chaban's case, she asks:

- What is it that you want to see happen?
- What is it you don't want to see happen?

- What would it look like if you arrived at a place that gave bad/poor care or bad/poor service?
- What would have to happen to take your humanity away – what would be unbearable, horrible, or torturous for you? [This last question is an uncommon one but unlocks some of people's biggest fears about the road ahead. Dr. Chaban worked with many Holocaust survivors so this question, in that context, is not as hard to imagine as you might think. Most of us have seen or experienced things that we never want to see or experience again.]

This begins a process of inquiry, as Dr. Chaban calls it. It helps her see what she needs to know to help her clients. They often do not know what they want or need in the beginning but the conversation starts a discussion that gets at their values and beliefs.

Determining their worst-case scenario

is to begin to practice preventive care. Once this is integrated in the care plan, the team has something to avoid. This is harm reduction and risk management in care. It helps us start to map out care, not simply tasks or protocols for treatment.

If you have an advisor, their role is to be helpful and supportive rather than to take charge and tell you what you should want and need. Their goal is to lead by example rather than tell you what to do. Over time, you may not need their support as often because your own confidence and skills increase.

Planning

As with all good planning, you think about what you will do in different situations before they happen. Just as we plan our fire escape routes from our homes, we can also know how to navigate any system and negotiate the best services possible. Thinking things through in advance and having a plan already in place will allow you to act naturally and with relative calm when the situation arises.

The model we recommend is:

Think about potential navigation situations regarding your health, finances, legal concerns, and other needs. You know you will use the healthcare systems over your lifetime. You will also need to make insurance claims, resolve any financial issues with your bank, and perhaps even have to be a witness in a court trial.

Talk with your family and friends about possible options of who can help with what as you should consider navigating these systems, negotiating the best services possible, and mediating difficulties if they arise.

Plan how to navigate, negotiate, and mediate and what resources to use.

Practice whatever skills you need to meet your specific needs. This may include improving communication skills, researching information on the internet, or taking workshops in financial planning, time management, or organizing information.

A plan starts with a simple listing of what you need, what you want and what you do not want to happen. If you followed the process above as described by Dr. Chaban, you will already have a detailed list of these things. For a simple, starting plan, you would break down your more complete plan into manageable steps.

Writing out this simple list allows everyone to come back to it to make sure that actions will help achieve the plan. As you progress through the navigation, negotiation and mediation process, you plan may change your plan.

For example, a healthcare list:

- I need excellent pain and symptom control.
- I want my family involved at all stages of my treatment
- I do not want to be in hospital any longer than necessary. I want to be at home as much as possible.

An education list for a parent whose son is having difficulty adjusting to Grade 9 may look like this based on a plan the parent is discussing with a vice-principal:

- I need a teacher, counselor or vice-principal to help my son acquire the skills to learn how to study almost anything with confidence. Once he can do that, all academics are open to him.
- I want a teacher, counselor or vice-principal to mentor my son to enjoy a rich balance of academics and extra-curricular activities (e.g., sports, theatre, music, art, interest clubs) which will add to his

confidence.

- I do not want the school to pre-determine what my son should study.

A financial list discussed with a financial planner:

- I need sufficient funds (60% current after-tax income) at age 65 to retire with my wife and two adult children (and their families potentially).
- I want to be able to create a plan now that will not require much decision making in the future – for example, automatic withdrawals into an RRSP while I am with my current employer.
- I do not want to take high risk with my investments – so investments in guaranteed funds so that no principle is lost.

The Single Thing a Family Caregiver or Advisor Can Do Better Than Anyone

Advisors or family caregivers are the only people who can take the time (often hours over many days) to identify what a person needs. Most service providers do not have the time or inclination to discover all aspects of what a person needs. They concentrate on one or two things they can offer a patient without looking at the whole person. Family caregivers and advisors, at their best, do exactly that – take the time to look at the whole person and all of their needs together.

Many people do not speak well, or speak a different language, or are unable to speak at all. How do they identify what they need? Even when we know what a person needs, finding the service or program that meets that need often takes a lot of time.

Sometimes you will need your family caregivers to help with a few things or teach you how to do a few things for yourself. These small differences can measurably enhance your life. .

Once the needs are determined, you begin to figure out who will help get the needs fulfilled, in what place, and by when. There are many options for meeting the needs (neighbors helping out, paid support, a nursing home) and the agreement about who does what makes it easier to develop a plan. The people involved may change very often depending on the time frame (a neighbor can help for a couple of weeks but often not for several years). Depending on the availability of friends and family, there may actually be very little service required in order to support the situation.

Navigation CHART

Once we know what you want, you can begin looking at how to meet these needs.

navCare's underlying philosophy is to never replace natural supports with systemic ones.

Simply put, if you, a family caregiver, friend, or neighbor can do something, then do not replace them with a paid person whose duty, time and loyalty belong to a service agency rather than to you.

The first approach, therefore, is to see how your needs can be met within the network of family, friends, neighbors, and others.

For the rest of this section, we will look only at what specific needs require outside help and which system(s) can provide that care or service.

Excellent navigators take a step-by-step approach to navigation. They begin with what you need and want that cannot be met by your own personal network of family, friends, neighbors, and others. They create a list of services you may need and a list of questions they want answered. The following chart summarizes this step-by-step process. Following the chart is a more detailed explanation.

Always keep detailed records so that over time you will develop your own list of favorite contacts and websites to check for information.

Resources for Information and Services			
People You Know	*Websites*	*Books/ Magazines*	*Organi-zations*
Family, friends, neighbors, co-workers, with specific skill sets or networks	Sites you trust and go to first including blogs, or newsletters, chat groups	Ones you trust and go to first (reference books), brochures & pamphlets	helplines, online chats, libraries, places that have info & services
Professionals you know & their staff:	Referral sites: 211, 311	Bookstores, online stores and libraries	
People You Do Not Know Yet	Official websites, then critical ones		
Professionals & their staff, bureaucrats, elders, information services (e.g. 211, 311, *Ask Elizabeth*)			

Strangers you meet randomly at parties, meetings, while waiting somewhere

Let us break down the chart's resources one by one by column.

Column 1: People You Know

Family and friends typically come first. Then you can look wider through your network including the people within your telephone or contact list. Your address book may have all the information you need to get what you want. Use it. Either your contacts will have information or they will know people who can be helpful. Once you have your plan of what you need and want, and your questions ready, it is time to let those people know you are looking for information.

Professionals & Staff You Know

These are your doctors, dentists, lawyers, pharmacists, accountants, and their support staff. Everyone you know and meet is a potential source of information or referrals. Learn from everyone including the maintenance, and secretarial staff that work with your professionals. The more important the information you need, the more people you need to connect with in your network.

People You Do Not Know

These are the professionals and their staff, bureaucrats, information services, and others you will meet during any navigation of a system. Some will be helpful. Some will not. All deserve a friendly approach. They may see dozens, if not many dozens of people during a day. To get what you need from them, you must stand out in some way and one of the best ways is to be pleasant, courteous, and ready with specific questions so you do not waste their time. You need to be precise and take up as little of their time as possible. Your attitude must be quite different from the other people they meet that day.

One useful starting phrase may be: "I only ask for seven minutes of your time to discuss…." This tells the person that you value their time and that after seven minutes they can expect the conversation to end. Typically, we ask for 10 minutes of someone's time. That then extends to 15 or 20 minutes. By picking an odd number, you are more likely to have their total focus.

These conversations may also take place with telephone operators or service representatives at help centers such as Telehealth – **1.866.797.0000** (nurses who answer questions about your specific healthcare need) or **211** operators (just dial 211 on your telephone) who have detailed lists of community and healthcare resources in your area. Again, your attitude can make their day. You may only have to navigate a system for a few hours, a few days, or a few weeks. They have to work in it for decades and many of their conversations may not be nice.

Strangers

Many people have told us that they have received very useful information from a conversation with a stranger while traveling or waiting in line somewhere. This does not mean talking with everyone you meet about your situation, but casual conversations often lead to whatever is most important for someone at the time. One person recounted how a passing physician, not related to their care in an emergency department, stopped and, after looking at him for a few seconds, said, "I know what's wrong with you." That physician was right and all the others involved in his care over 10 previous years had been wrong in their diagnoses. This was random luck, yet it was only possible because the person was open to talking about their condition with a stranger—in this case, a very knowledgeable one.

Column 2: Websites

If you want specific information, you can start with websites you already trust. Our References section lists ones that have been proven reliable. These may include general reference sites such as the 211 website for your geographic region. This site lists healthcare, community, and social service agencies in your community.

Another level of websites is the "official" website of whatever system you need to navigate, whether that is the school board for your region or the disease-specific organization that provides supports to clients and their families.

Type the name of the organization or disease/condition into your browser to locate the official website. Do a quick check of all the materials and services available there.

Before getting into too much detail, search for websites that support the official website's content and programs and other websites that are critical. For example, in the case of the school board, check any parent groups, community groups, or student groups to see what they have to say about the subject you are researching. If you want to find out about services for your child who needs extra support that your school does not offer, check the official school board website but also student helplines.

In other words, do not rely solely on any single website for your answers. A good journalist must get at least three sources for any information they want to publish. You should also look for at least three sources of information before you make important decisions.

This would be just as true for investment or banking information as it is for healthcare or legal information. The homework needs to be done.

A way to evaluate services is to see what measures a system uses. Although not always easily found on an official website, a search through your browser for "balanced scorecard AND name of system" can be interesting. For example, type in "balanced scorecard AND your local hospital" to see what information the hospital collects.

You can also type in "critique" or "complaint" AND "name of system" into your browser to find complaints against a specific system. For example: "complaint AND name of your local school board" can lead you to useful sites. Follow links to other credible critical sites to go deeper into a system.

Column 3: Books, Magazines, Brochures, and Pamphlets

Sometimes you need some background information to help you understand something more specific. For example, there are many excellent books and magazines on financial planning. These are good to review before looking for specific investment tools like retirement or education savings plans, stock market investments, or government bonds.

Brochures and pamphlets can also provide you with specific questions you should ask anyone you talk with while navigating a system. Many excellent brochures or books on family caregiving give specific examples of the types of questions you might ask before agreeing to a test or treatment.

For example, www.carelibrary.com offers free online books on caregiving, home care, hospice palliative care, and communication skills.

Start with books and magazines you already trust. Then look in bookstores, in person or online (e.g., amazon.com), for books on your topic of interest or for an author you trust. Also look for brochures, pamphlets, and other shorter printed materials that could be helpful. Many professional offices have such information in their waiting rooms.

In libraries and bookstores, it can also help to see what books are shelved near the one you are looking for. Researchers often find the best materials are actually the books near the one they thought would be best. Browsing the shelves is an excellent research method.

Column 4: Organizations

Aside from navigating within a specific system, there are many organizations that provide information, referrals, and supports that can also be helpful. For example, during your research you may find a disease-specific organization and decide to visit their local office. There you may discover they have written material beyond what is available on their website as well as staff and volunteers who can answer your questions in a more relaxed way than someone on the telephone. This is an opportunity to start nurturing working relationships with one or two of the staff or volunteers.

You may also find they have support groups for people who are experiencing a similar situation as you are. These support groups are helpful in many ways, one of the most important of which is providing an opportunity for people to compare notes on what is working for them and what is not. It can be helpful to share a coffee or connect through social media with some of the members of such a group to find out more about what they have learned.

Next Steps

You have your plans, your questions, and your research. What's next?

- Journalist Standard When reviewing materials, analyze your research like a journalist would. A journalist cannot report something as fact unless they have three reliable sources. This can be your guide to ensuring that what you are getting from the internet is reliable.
- Choose Priorities You cannot do everything at once. Pick the most important next steps based on what is most likely to move you toward fulfilling your information and planning needs. Many people use a 1-2-3 priority system: #1 is assigned to those things that should be done first, #2 for things that can wait a short time, and #3 for things that can wait several weeks or months.

We spend 80% of our time accomplishing 20% of our work. We need to reverse the order so we spend 20% of our time accomplishing 80% of our work. Effective time management can be very helpful here. This is not for emergency situations but for when you have time to create a plan and then implement it.

In real situations, this means that talking with a knowledgeable person is likely to get better results than surfing the internet for days on end. You may be more comfortable searching the internet than you are talking with strangers, but getting through your discomfort and building up the confidence that comes with practice will save you hours of research.

Taking Notes

Not all of us enjoy writing notes about telephone calls, office appointments, and the like. However, it is one of the best ways to stick to your priorities and to find the shortcuts to whatever you need. If you keep everything in your head, especially when you are under stress, you will miss important information, forget about an appointment or task, and easily get sidetracked to avoid working on the big things. So take notes.

You can create your own note system or use the one at the end of this book. Keep things together in a single notebook or file or, best of all, a binder. This will allow you to keep everything together, move pages around as you need them, and remove pages when you need to take them to an appointment or consult them when making your telephone calls.

Final Steps

You will go through the planning, research, appointments, meetings, treatments, and telephone calls for what feels like forever. You will go back to your contact list. You will continue to research on the internet and in the library. You will go back to organizations and support groups until you do not need them anymore.

It will be a roller coaster ride of successes and failures, joys and frustrations.

Persistence and a dogged commitment to do what is needed to get the best services possible is the number one characteristic of successful advisors and navigators. That does not mean there will not be times when you will want to quit or strike out in anger. It does mean you will have a better than average chance of getting what you want. Always return to the main goals. Do not lose sight of what you are trying to accomplish.

Navigation is a relatively straightforward process that, unfortunately, takes too much time, too much research, and too much energy. It should be a lot easier. Some systems are making it simpler.

We go back to basics to help us manage this task:

- Think about what you need and who can provide you some of the information. People are faster than computers when they know the inside information about how to navigate a system.
- Talk to as many people as you need to so you feel comfortable beginning the navigation process and taking it to its successful completion.
- Plan how to tackle big or complex navigation processes.
- Practice successful navigation techniques using some of the resources in this manual, and the other *navCare* books and binders, to

keep track of the information you are collecting.

- Lastly, share what you learn. You are becoming an expert on navigating a specific system. Make some notes about what worked and what did not. Note who was particularly helpful and who was not. Then, let people in your circle of family and friends know you would like to help them navigate the same or similar systems.

Negotiation

Negotiating is simply talking to people in a clear way about what you need and how they might help.

It is about respecting their time. Keep your conversations short and to the point. Practice so that you can say what you need to in less than 7 minutes.

Negotiating is about being assertive when people are not listening, without being rude.

It is following the golden rule of treating people as you want to be treated.

Negotiating is about standing up for yourself or a loved one.

We negotiate all the time. When we talk with friends about what movie we want to see, it is a negotiation because rarely does everyone want to watch the same movie. When a couple is deciding where to eat dinner, it is a negotiation. When children ask to borrow the car, it is a negotiation.

Some negotiations are very quick and others take some time.

The following information will help you negotiate better in all kinds of situations.

Negotiation is a constant process through which you, your family, and service providers work together using good communication skills to achieve the best services possible. The intent is always a cooperative, collaborative approach to meet or surpass the typical benchmark for excellence.

When negotiating with people within a system you can keep two things in mind:

1. What do you want from them to help you meet your needs?
2. What do they need from you to feel good about their work?

It is helpful in negotiations to understand the various roles played by the different negotiators. Systems want to save money, reduce staff time, and become more efficient. Those systems that need to compete for your business are easiest to deal with.

Those that do not need you will find it easier to dismiss your wishes, concerns, and questions. Their priority may be to get paperwork done before the end of the shift or to reduce overall costs to make their boss appreciate their efforts. If you can help them do that while meeting your needs you will have found the magic balance of an effective negotiation.

Your role or that of your family caregivers is to:

- Get the proper information to the person within the system with whom you are dealing.
- Understand the system from the inside out as best as you can. This will involve some homework up

front, talking with people you know within the system and, perhaps, doing some internet research.

- Evaluate information received.
- Review alternatives and choose the best option in your circumstances or understand what is on offer and then regroup or redefine the next step.
- Give the best possible personal information clearly and as briefly as possible, perhaps even in writing. Your professional care providers can read faster than you can talk, but keep it to less than one page.
- Communicate honestly about your physical, emotional, spiritual, and information needs.
- When possible, learn to use prayer, mindfulness meditation, and/or visualization techniques to reduce your anxiety and stress. You will be easier to talk with if you are less anxious.
- Follow decisions made together

with your advisor, your family, and those involved with you in the system, or explain why you choose not to at this time.

In order to fulfill your roles and achieve the most success possible in any given situation, you need excellent communication skills. The following is information mostly for advisors and telephone/online coaches. You can pick out specific techniques to pass along to a client or family as needed. They need you to be the expert. They can improve their skills once they have more time.

Communication Skills

The word "communication" comes from the root word "common." It is about speaking a common language that is easily understood by all participants in a conversation. The following are a few techniques that can help improve your communication skills:

- Acknowledge (repeat back, paraphrase) feelings versus "topping" the other person's story with one of your own experiences. For example, if a doctor tells you during a visit that they are very busy, tell them you understand rather than telling them how busy you are. You are there to get their help, not compete to see who is busier.
- Know the other person's name and help them remember yours.
- Understand mutual stresses and help others understand your particular stresses right now.
- Pay attention to words and body language. If someone is ignoring you or avoiding looking at you, ask them politely to slow down for a moment and speak to you directly.
- Use a person's name the way you normally do (e.g. Mrs. Jacobs, the accountant, should not become Sue, dear, or honey just because you

want her help.) Maintain the social distance you have kept in the past unless the person wants a change.

- Encourage family meetings to help make important decisions.
- Encourage a single spokesperson for you and your family so that care providers do not have to communicate the same information three different times to three different family members.

Resolving Problems

When trying to resolve a problem with a particular person in a particular system, a quick tip can be bringing in another person from within the system. For example, in health care, that might be a nurse, chaplain, social worker, physician, or supervisor. In the education system, it might be a vice-principal or a social worker. In the legal system, it might be the Duty Counsel or the supervisor of the Crown Attorney.

Refer to the chapter on mediation for more detailed suggestions.

Service Providers' Lament

Service providers often feel they do not have enough time. They may say: "I don't have enough time to communicate the way you want me to."

We spend 70% of our waking hours communicating. Therefore, we have to use our time effectively. If we were to spend only a fraction of our daily communication time communicating better, we could avoid some simple, yet sometimes deadly, misunderstandings. Poor communication in health care can lead to unnecessary tests, medication errors, inadequate pain management, or simply bad feelings between people. In the legal system it can lead to someone being convicted of a crime they did not commit because people did not listen and/or the client could not communicate properly. In the insurance business, it can lead to a claim taking many months to resolve rather than a few weeks.

Good communicators can say, "ten minutes with me is like 50 minutes with someone else." And it's true!

As we have discussed, there are other forms of communication besides talking. Using body language, a touch, a smile, or a look of concern and empathy to show genuine interest can shorten many conversations by getting right to the important issues.

Difficulties

People have a personal history including those you want to help you meet your needs. They may have family problems, be in an abusive relationship, work too many hours without enough sleep, or be in physical pain because of a chronic health condition.

Yes, they are supposed to leave their personal life at home, but few of us are capable of doing that. So, in your negotiation with others, just be alert to the fact that although your situation is critical to you, it may not be critical for them. It is not fair. But if you know this, your communication style may be more relaxed, more respectful, and more thoughtful.

In emergency situations, of course, you won't have time to be this thoughtful, but most of our negotiations in life do not take place during emergency situations.

You cannot change people. You can offer help and understanding when there is time and opportunity. You can expect excellence without demanding it in every situation. You can be understanding without putting your own needs last.

Negotiation is about two or more people or organizations achieving their own objectives through a change in their relationship. It is about getting the best possible deal for yourself while trying to ensure that the other people get as much as possible of what they need and want as well. Effective negotiations ensure a long-lasting working relationship.

Negotiation at its simplest is an easily understood process but one that takes continuous practice to perfect. Negotiation at higher levels and in matters of life and death should not be done lightly. People's beliefs run deep and negotiators are apt to run into distrust and strong emotions if assumptions are made or values are not understood. In addition, when the stakes are high, such as when deciding which healthcare treatment is best, which supervisor or manager to negotiate with, or how to lodge a complaint within a system, you may use negotiation strategies that are meant to dominate or win over the other party. These only work once or twice. To build a long-term relationship, you need to negotiate in a more mutually beneficial way.

Negotiators need to be highly skilled. It is helpful to ask, "Is there anything you think I need to know that I have not asked about?" This way, everyone gives their best and most authentic input.

The Basic Skills You Need

The successful negotiator has the following abilities in their bag of skills.

Basic Communication Skills

Good verbal and written communication skills can help you make your points easy to understand so that you have a better chance of getting what you need. You do not need a university degree to communicate well. Basic communication skills means the ability to speak or write in short, clear sentences — to get your ideas across to others quickly.

Understanding

Understanding someone's viewpoints and needs is not the same as approving of them. Countries constantly negotiate treaties even though their basic philosophies are different. The purpose of understanding someone else is not just to gain a negotiation tool, but also to take the approach of negotiating **with** someone rather than **against** someone.

Predictable, Fair, Firm

If you are predictable in your behavior, fair with your family and friends, and firm in keeping your commitments to others, then people will be able to trust you even when they strongly disagree with you.

Acceptance

You may strongly disagree with a person's behavior or ideas without having to strongly dislike their personality, culture, or beliefs. Such an acceptance may allow you to persuade people (over time) that your viewpoints are equally valid and worth their time to listen to and understand. Persuasion has longer lasting results than forcing someone to do things your way.

Everyday Negotiations

Negotiation is an everyday occurrence if you live with others in your home. For example, you need to work out who uses the bathroom and when, who does which chores, what happens during emergencies, and so much more.

Negotiations take time and when they

are done well they may result in better services, products and relationships.

Here are a few tips:

- Spend time actively listening and understanding (*really* understanding) what the other person wants.
- Look at some alternatives beyond the normal ones you typically generate.
- Agree on something that is fair to everyone.
- Make sure that your agreement also helps the long-term relationship you may have with the other person.

Beyond these basics there are many strategies that we will look at later in this material. The important point in everyday negotiations is not to harm the other person or yourself, or to let anyone else harm you. Mutual respect and mutual benefits are what lead to long-term negotiating successes.

Strategies

Strategies are tools you can use to change a situation, including the important elements of timing, location, and the specific techniques of negotiation.

Different strategies are helpful in different situations. Consider both the short-term objectives and the long-term effects of any strategy. If you plan to work together with the people for any length of time you must understand the long-term consequences of the negotiation for your working relationship. Mend bridges whenever possible rather than destroying relationships for short-term gains. This is true with your bank teller, your children's teachers, regular bus driver, and neighbors.

Expect Disagreement, Conflict, and Tension

Many negotiations reach a point

where people begin to think that they have wasted their time and there is no hope of reaching an agreement. This is usually the most important time to review and take stock of what points you have already agreed to, what criteria for success have been identified, what interests you have in common, and what areas you can choose to disagree on without losing the opportunity to reach some kind of effective and amicable agreement.

Asking Questions

Good communication tools, such as asking genuine, open-ended questions, encourage people to negotiate in good faith. Used as a technique to get your way, this strategy will fail. Used as a genuine means of understanding the other person's needs and interests, this strategy will inspire a negotiating environment of mutual gain.

Avoidance

You can either delay or avoid negotiating or taking any action. You can use this strategy to provide you (and perhaps others) time to develop a clearer plan. You can use this to allow time for people to express their anger, re-evaluate differing positions, allow the problem to remain until it changes by itself, or accept the situation as it is.

The Unexpected

Sometimes doing the unexpected will help others see your point of view differently while you maintain your negotiating objectives. You can either do something that brings you closer to others' ways of thinking or take an opposite approach to highlight areas of differences. For example, imagine that you are negotiating with a receptionist about your next appointment. Each time you go through this process, there is frustration as your schedule is not easily adapted to theirs. One day, unexpectedly, you show up with a small bouquet of flowers with a note that says, "I appreciate how frustrating scheduling can be. Thank you for always trying to meet my scheduling needs." If done genuinely, your working relationship with the receptionist will improve. People respect someone who understands how hard their job really is.

I Win

You can (if you have the power) direct people without accepting any room for negotiation. This strategy works in emergencies or in smaller disagreements where people do not have the energy to reach a negotiated settlement. This strategy is not effective for any long-term changes you may want to make.

Leave

Sometimes it is necessary to leave a negotiation for either a short time or a longer time. The timing depends on your power or influence and the type of negotiation you are involved in. Leaving may also signal that you accept a portion, or all, of a settlement but that you continue to disagree with the decision-making process. Unless you follow up with some changes to improve the situation and clarify your concerns, the end result will not satisfy anyone.

One Person Leaves, Another One Remains

Sometimes it is necessary for one or several team members to exit a negotiation but leave one person behind to indicate commitment to resolving the negotiating issues. When some people leave, it implies you have some negotiating strengths and the timing can permit people to re-examine their perspectives.

One Thing at a Time

Try to limit your negotiations to one or two items at a time. Trying to accomplish too much at once reduces the chances of being effective and getting results that are mutually agreeable. Use your communication skills to keep your stories, requests, and negotiations short. No one really needs to hear the whole story – just the relevant pieces.

Compare to Similar Situations

Sometimes advance research will reveal situations similar to the one you are presently negotiating where people received the level of service you want. These other situations may provide you with statistics about possible successes or difficulties. The situations can be internal, external, or, if possible, both. Your research will also provide you useful information and, therefore, credibility as a professional willing to go the extra mile to resolve a situation to everyone's benefit.

Mix and Match

Sometimes it is useful to use several strategies at once to increase the possibility of success and to allow others to choose strategies they are more comfortable with.

Role of Dimes

A role of 50 dimes equals $5.00. Sometimes it is easier to ask for several dimes at a time rather than the whole $5.00. Even within one negotiation you can get commitment to smaller portions of your wants and needs and increase your requests a bit at a time to get to the point you really want. It may be a little more time-consuming but it can get you the results and commitment you want. This is helpful as you build a long-term relationship with someone you will have to deal with for many years.

Bottom Line Limits

Some aspects of your negotiation may

involve issues or items that are non-negotiable for ethical, economic, or organizational reasons. Be clear about them in order to indicate your level of commitment and power over these points. For example, if you typically have to wait more than 30 minutes in the waiting room to see your doctor, lawyer, or accountant, ask to be called or texted 10 minutes before the person is ready to see you so that you can go do something else nearby while waiting. Some pharmacies and car dealerships, for example, give clients a pager that buzzes when they are ready for you, allowing you to continue to shop or go for a coffee break.

Time Out

Time out is asking for a few minutes, hours, or days to discuss options with your family and supporters. If you need to make a decision about treatments in a hospital, or during a court case or when negotiating special services for your child in school, you may need time to examine the options more carefully before deciding. Tell people how long you expect to take before getting back to them with your decision.

Giving Up Some Control

Sometimes it is very useful to allow others to take some control over the negotiation to symbolize your trust in them or your willingness to meet them halfway. You can also use this strategy to offer others a range of choices and give them the responsibility of choosing the next move.

Dirty Tricks

When someone uses intimidation, lies, psychological abuse, or other pressure tactics there are several things you can do. Often people react by ignoring this illegal, unethical, or uncomfortable behavior in the hope that it will go away or that ignoring it will help the negotiation end in success. Other people fight back in similar ways and the negotiation turns out to be a battle of wills and ill-conceived strategies.

It is more effective to recognize the tactic as unfair, tell the other negotiators that you have recognized the inappropriate tactic, and ask them why they feel the tactic is legitimate or helpful. Again, concentrate on the procedures used rather than who used them. Often just speaking about what you think is happening, in a non-threatening way, takes the power out of the tactic and allows the negotiators to get back to the real problems being negotiated.

The Squeaky Wheel

Many of us have heard the expression, "The squeaky wheel gets the grease." It refers to a bike or car wheel that makes a noise and needs grease to silence it. In everyday life it refers to the idea that people who complain get better results than people who quietly accept poor or negligent care.

The choice is whether to ask for help in a positive, assertive manner or a loud and disrespectful one. Again, the positive, assertive way typically gets better long-term results.

One technique that works for successful negotiators is to ask a front-line person *quietly and calmly*: "Who do I yell at to get *you* what you need to help my loved one?"

This may sound counter to our motto of nurturing relationships. However, as one negotiator described it, when he used this technique to ask nurses who he needed to yell at to get them what they needed to help his father, they smiled and dialed the telephone for him. They felt supported by his taking on a more assertive advocacy role as their hands were tied by poor internal communications at a higher level. When he got on the phone he found out he was speaking with the Director of Nurses. He repeated the phrase "Who do I yell at to get you what you need to help my father?" He could hear her calm and patient response that she was not upset but ready to help her staff help his father. She said, "Oh, you don't need to yell at anyone Sir. We'll get your father into ICU immediately where he can get what he needs."

Note, that at no time did the negotiator yell. Although he was at his limit watching his father go through painful and debilitating seizures because of brain cancer, he asked the nurses who were trying their best, who he should speak to. The word "yell" is usually inappropriate, but when one's limit is reached, it can be a useful technique to advocate on behalf of front-line professionals who cannot advocate as strongly as a family member can. They felt supported -- not intimidated.

Writing Things Out

Too often negotiations get bogged down in uncertainty and frustration because you have not clearly written out what you need. Emotions can run high especially when situations are very serious. Writing things out means you will not forget what it is you are negotiating for. Keep your list of needs down to three at each phase of the negotiation so it is easy to measure if the need is met. Once a need is met, you can add something else to the list. Asking for too much at once means you will likely lose the ability to evaluate what has been done and what still needs doing.

Summary

- Negotiation is an everyday act and many of us enjoy the give and take of negotiating with family, friends, and colleagues.
- Negotiation is about changing a relationship between two or more people or organizations. It is about

getting the best possible services and care for yourself while trying to ensure that the other people get as much of what they need and want as well to ensure a long-lasting working relationship.

- Negotiation for some people is a game that you win when you get most or everything that you want regardless of what the other people get. For others, negotiation is a process of finding out what everyone needs and coming up with the best alternative to help them fulfill those needs. The second alternative has a longer success rate over months and years.
- Regardless of which view you take, negotiations involve preparation, working closely with other people, agreeing to a specific course of action, and understanding what your own strengths and learning needs are so you can ask an advisor or family caregiver to help with the negotiation.

Your Notes on Navigation

Mediation

You will likely experience difficulties as you navigate and negotiate to the best services and care possible in all systems.

Whenever you are part of a large system, either as a customer or as a worker, there will be inevitable difficulties in communication and service delivery. This is only natural. The complexities of large systems may result in excellent services most of the time, but not all of the time.

Sometimes it is a communication problem. Other times it is a misunderstanding of what is possible and what is not possible in a given circumstance. Most people want to resolve difficulties quickly, calmly, and effectively. Sometimes the difficulty is between the person and their providers. More often it is between professionals (the major source of stress in health care is interdisciplinary conflicts or conflicts within the same discipline).

The following material covers the key skill set in mediation: resolving conflicts.

There are many other skill sets that might help, such as time and stress management. If you visit the website www.carelibrary.com you will find a free online book titled *Practical Leadership*. This book is designed specifically for leadership and improved skills development for healthcare providers, but most of the skills are generic for people navigating, negotiating, and mediating in any system. There are chapters on time and stress management, assertive communication, team building, running effective meetings, and much more. All are free for reading online or you can print any sections that may be helpful.

Introduction

This section is quite general in scope because there are just too many aspects of a conflict to go into much detail here. Use the general skills described here in your specific situation. Adapt them to meet your needs. Bring in others such as your family, friends, and advisors to help you decide which of the following strategies or skills might be most helpful in your circumstances.

How do you resolve conflicts? There are several questions that must be asked first:

- Does everyone involved recognize that a conflict exists or is it just you who wants someone else to change their ways?
- If everyone involved recognizes that a conflict exists, are they as **committed** as you to resolving that conflict? If not, you will need to find something that the other

person will see as a benefit to them in order to get their commitment to help you resolve the conflict.

- Is someone else causing the conflict or are you also a part of that conflict? Conflict is usually not a one-sided problem.
- Do you recognize that you resolve problems for yourself first and for other people second? In other words, to resolve conflicts to your own satisfaction, you need to do it for yourself first. This will be particularly hard for the "peacemakers" in families and workplaces who usually resolve conflicts by giving in to others' demands in order to keep the peace, rather than making the effort needed to resolve conflicts to everyone's satisfaction.
- Do you recognize that you always have control over how you respond to a conflict and that sometimes your response includes making small changes versus big ones **or**

making the decision to leave the situation yourself?

Whether conflicts are large or small you must understand that other people are not going to change their personalities or behaviors just to please you. Other people must believe there are clear benefits for them in changing just as you have to believe that changes you make will benefit you. Anyone who changes their personality or behavior just to please someone else will usually become bitter about those changes over time.

There will always be personality differences between people that can cause difficulties. **People will not (and often, cannot) change their basic personalities.** (Ask newlyweds who thought their spouse would change their habits for them out of love.) Since personality conflicts will always exist we must concentrate on looking at specific behaviors people use rather than evaluating their personalities.

Behaviors can be changed or modified if the other person knows how they affect you. When all is said and done, you will not like everyone you encounter. There is no reason that you have to. You should be able to respect or at least tolerate most people and still achieve a satisfactory outcome.

The following is some general background information on what can cause conflict, the types of conflict, and specific methods to help resolve them.

You may be thinking: **"All this information is wonderful but it just won't work in my case. I've tried everything but they just won't change. I'm powerless."**

People are not powerless. We always have the power to choose how we respond. Other people cannot make us happy or unhappy, angry or sad. If we have a conflict with someone and we have tried everything we can to resolve that conflict in good faith (a key element), then we have some choices:

- Evaluate whether the conflict is a mutual problem between you and the other person(s) **or** is it really a problem that only you can deal with.
- If the other person is not willing to make any effort to resolve the problem, can you:
  - ignore them and make the best of it?
  - bring in other people to help you resolve the issue (e.g., a social worker in healthcare or education systems)?
  - go to a person in higher authority to see if the problem can be resolved there?

Viktor Frankl, a survivor of the Nazi concentration camps lost his family during the Holocaust. He said that regardless of what horrors were inflicted on him during those years, no one was ever able to dictate to him how he must respond. How he responded to these most difficult of situations was always under his control. He has used that practical philosophy to help people make real changes in their lives.

Frankl understood that sometimes you cannot change the circumstances you face because of major systemic problems. However, you can control how you respond to the circumstances and make small changes to make such severe situations more tolerable. People can often still laugh, cry, join together, use their memories of the past, make their plans for the future, and use their inner strength to help themselves in these situations.

In the less severe situations that we often face we can certainly do many of the same things, as well as develop the love of our families and friends and use a clear-headed analysis of what is really happening to us to make the changes we need to maintain control over our lives and our feelings.

In the day-to-day conflicts that we face and with the foresight to imagine how we will evaluate these situations 10 years from now, we can put our conflicts into perspective and decide how hard and for how long we will try to resolve the conflicts before moving on to greater challenges.

Ten years from now, whatever stresses or conflicts you experience as part of your navigation of systems and negotiating for better services and care will be mostly forgotten. The day-to-day stresses and conflicts that are inherent in being part of a large system will be forgotten. What you will remember are the results, both positive and negative, a few specific joyful experiences, and a few specific difficult and stressful ones.

The following tools will help you to minimize the negative memories you will carry with you and enhance the likelihood of creating and remembering moments of joy, relief, acceptance, and love.

The principle of using your conflict resolution skills effectively is to **participate actively** in the process, **organize** your skills, **persist** during difficult times, and be **creative**. The more effectively we use our skills, the more time we will have to enjoy other parts of our lives.

Conflict Can Be Useful

Conflict can be useful if:

- results in solutions to problems
- helps people to understand themselves and others better
- helps us discover new and important issues
-
- helps us to communicate more honestly and openly with others
- helps us to get rid of some of our anger, anxiety, and fear resulting in a more adaptable and flexible

personality
- helps people to work better together
- helps people to develop their personalities and skills to ever increasing heights of personal satisfaction
- helps people to examine, and potentially revise, their life's priorities

Conflict Can Be Destructive

Conflict can be destructive if:

- drains us of our physical and mental energies
- causes us to concentrate on complaining and ridiculing people we disagree with and who we won't make an effort to understand
- reduces co-operation between people
- causes us to think badly about ourselves and others and encourages us to have a poorer self-

image
- detracts us from working on our primary goals or purposes
- taints the environment we are in and reduces our enjoyment of others
- carries over to negatively influence our personal and home lives.

Conflict Resolution Strategies

There are various strategies for resolving conflicts. Depending on the specific situation and with whom you have the conflict, you will use some strategies more often than others. In fact, we often are less likely to resolve conflicts with family members than with colleagues because we assume family is forever and doesn't require as much effort as our work relationships.

Avoiding Conflict

We use this strategy when we think the issue is not worth fighting about or if we deny there is a problem. You need to pick your opportunities to resolve really important conflicts and accept that minor conflicts are not worth your energy right now. For example, arguing over a parking spot at the hospital, court house, or insurance company is probably not a good use of your time when you are facing a major illness, court case, or insurance claim.

We may avoid important issues because we are afraid of hurting someone's feelings or because we just "can't be bothered." When this happens, we cannot blame the other person for the conflict remaining unresolved. People cannot read our minds. If they do not know the conflict is important to us, they will continue to behave as they always have.

Giving In

We may use this strategy when it is easier to give in than to spend time resolving the conflict. We may be more passive than others or bored with trying to smooth things out. We may also be afraid of conflict or disharmony and, therefore, always give in to "keep everyone happy." This strategy is also effective when we deem the issue as one that we can "let go of" without harming our relationship with the person.

Win/Lose

Children often think their parents follow this strategy: "I'm the parent so you have to do what I say." It is similar to people of different levels of authority in an organization or people who are more aggressive who say "Just do it!" This survival-of-the-fittest strategy may be very appropriate during an emergency situation when someone decides on everyone's behalf that they must exit a building during a fire. However, it is destructive in maintaining long-term working and personal relationships.

Compromising

Compromise does not mean that everyone is happy. Usually it is used when two people have extreme positions and agree to meet in the middle. Depending on how extreme the initial positions are, it is unlikely that either or both parties will be satisfied. Compromise is often used in political, economic, arms control, and management-labor negotiations. If the end result is just a compromise then the parties will leave dissatisfied and this dissatisfaction will make future negotiations even more difficult.

Problem-Solving

This is the most time-consuming and most rewarding strategy for resolving major and minor conflicts. In this strategy people are committed to making the effort to resolve the conflict. People listen to each other and use good communication skills to speak openly and honestly. People may not end the conflict liking each other, but they may respect the other person's commitment to their honestly-held beliefs and their willingness to discuss behavioral changes. This type of conflict resolution ends in a mutually agreed upon and beneficial solution without either party having to make major concessions. It is often called a win/ win strategy.

The potential for conflict while navigating systems and negotiating services is great because of: the constant need for communicating complex issues among people with different language skills; the need for many people to work together despite considerable systemic differences; differences in attitude, training, commitment, socio-economic background, and personal competencies; and the personality differences between people.

For example, a bureaucrat who has dedicated her life to her work clashes with a colleague who plans to quit as soon as a better paying job comes along. Their lack of mutual loyalty and respect may be a real source of the conflict. When you enter the picture, you may have just caught her after a heated disagreement with her colleague. She will regret not serving you well later but that does not diminish the fact that your needs were not met. When you return, it can be very helpful to start fresh rather than presume she is always someone with whom it is difficult to negotiate.

Another example might be that you may want to take your child out of class for a longer vacation time that is against school board policy. Any tests or assignments due will count as zero because your child is not there. However, you strongly believe that the child and the rest of your family will learn a great deal more by learning together (e.g., a trip to a rain forest, or an extended stay to help a grandparent who is ill). To problem-solve this situation you may come to a mutual agreement that the child will complete some homework or assignments while away and do make-up tests upon their return. Although still against the school board's policy, an exception is being made that fulfills the school's study requirements while allowing the family an experience they would otherwise miss.

Lastly, in health care, your great-aunt who is a nun is dying and you are trying to be helpful. She is adamant that she does not want to take pain control medications even though she knows her particular type of cancer will become very painful. Her physician is equally adamant that he does not want to see her suffer nor let his staff watch her suffer even if it means going against her wishes.

The problem-solving approach here might be to bring in a palliative care team that deals with dying patients daily. Their solution is for the patient to be allowed to continue to refuse treatment (as is the law) but that a) the patient be supported in a palliative care room within the hospital that is more soundproof and b) that your aunt's fellow nuns, family, and friends be given instruction on how to minimize the pain naturally. She will still experience the pain but in a more supportive environment than is typically possible in a hospital and where her fellow sisters are more comfortable allowing her to live her life fully until they die in their own way. There will be support for the extended family and care providers during and after your aunt's illness.

Preventing Conflict

The following are some techniques for preventing conflict:

- **Assume that everyone is doing the best they can with the knowledge they have at that time.** Few people get up in the morning with the sole purpose of their life being to make your life miserable. If something they do upsets you, assume that it was not intentional and try to talk to the person about it. Tell them how you feel when they do something specific. Talk about their behavior. Do not accuse them. Try to understand why they did something.

- **Use humor, laughter, and play**. Humor, laughter, and play bring people closer together. It is hard to dislike people with whom you spend time laughing. Laughter and smiling are contagious and encourage an environment where people can talk out problems with a sense of humor.
- **Communication skills**. Communication skills are critical to help us avoid and deal with conflicts. Communication is not a 50-50 type of thing. You each must give 100% to ensure that the other

person understands you and you understand them. You don't do this for someone else; you do it for yourself because it gives you control. Don't be afraid to ask questions to clarify anything the person has said.

- **Courtesy**. Courtesy is still the key to unlocking people's positive feelings. Saying "thank you," "please," “I forgive you,” and "would you please?" encourages people to respect you and others. Just as importantly, saying “I'm sorry,” “I was wrong,” or “Can I help?” helps bridge a gap between people. You can act as a role model to others who have forgotten the power of courtesy.
- **Participate**. People need to see you making an effort to make things easier for everyone. In health care it may mean getting something for yourself rather than expecting a nurse to do it for you. In education, it means showing that you

participate in your child's school activities.

- **Acknowledge people's successes and your mistakes**. A sincere compliment and acceptance of your own mistakes shows your honesty and your willingness to recognize excellence in other people. Be specific about whatever someone has done well so that your compliments do not appear superficial or like a public relations ploy. Also, avoid complimenting routine work as the other person may assume you are being rude. For example, imagine sitting in a waiting room and overhearing the receptionist on a call. "The way you answer the phone is very professional," may be interpreted by the person in this way: "I always answer the phone this way. What's the big deal? What does she want from me?"
- **People can be skeptical of kindness** in today's busy world.

That same compliment from you might be given this way, "I couldn't help overhearing how you helped that person on the phone who was clearly quite upset when they called. From what I could hear, you really calmed them down, found out what they needed, and helped them figure out how to get it. I can tell you from personal experience, what you just did will make that caller's day and she will tell her family and friends about how kind and helpful you were."

- **Do not argue with or criticize people in front of their colleagues**. Few things upset people more than being embarrassed in front of colleagues or the public. Always provide constructive criticism in private.
- **Personal rumors can hurt people**. As fascinating as they may be to listen to, you must recognize that the information is probably inaccurate. Do not repeat rumors

about people you know. If you respect other people's privacy they may do the same in return.

Dealing with Conflicts

- **Talk it out**. If someone does something that hurts you physically or emotionally, leave the situation and take some time to think clearly about what happened. Use this "cooling off" time to clearly identify and deal with your emotions. Identify the issues in the conflict and determine what you would like to change. Develop an approach to dealing with the conflict. Use "I" statements to tell the person clearly how you feel when they do something. For example, "I do not understand what I may have done to upset you so much that we cannot discuss possible outcomes for my client." When you have resolved the conflict, do not bring it up again in the future.

- **Get help**. Sometimes a conflict cannot be resolved by some of the strategies suggested in this material. Sometimes a third party, a supervisor, or another Advisor can help people communicate more clearly and specifically without some of the emotion that can cloud issues.
- **Ultimately, someone may have to leave**. If all the suggestions and strategies in this resource have been tried, and have failed, you may have to recognize that your only alternative is for you to get service elsewhere. If that is not possible, then going higher up the power structure may be necessary. As a last resort, you may need to hire a lawyer to act as your official advisor. A legal process can take a very long time but sometimes you have no other recourse. This is less effective in health care where issues need to be resolved more quickly (depending on your condition).

However, if legal action is necessary, get a lawyer with a great deal of experience in this type of situation. Just as you want a surgeon who has performed the same surgery many times, you want a lawyer who has worked with system abuses many times.

Hot Buttons

Hot buttons are personal triggers in us that cause us to react to other people's behaviors without thinking about what to do first. We may respond irrationally and powerfully. For example, someone has pushed your hot button if you react with instant anger when they call you a name you really dislike. Our brothers and sisters were very good at finding our hot buttons when we were children!

The assumption that many people have about hot buttons is that other people can control our behaviors. This is a belief that you can choose not to believe any more. You always have control over how you react to other people's words and behaviors. First, you must be aware of what causes immediate responses from you. Some examples of hot buttons are: being left on hold too long on the telephone; working with complicated telephone systems requiring you to input number after number to get to a message that is not very helpful; being asked to fill in yet another waiver form; waiting in long lineups; talking with people who look down on you because of a difference in culture or education; or dealing with disrespectful customer service representatives. One of the most common hot buttons is not getting a straight answer to a question.

Perhaps the most common hot button is being made to feel like your needs are your own fault and that you should feel lucky that someone will talk to you at all.

Determine what your hot buttons are and how to respond differently. If someone yells at you in public, you could leave and discuss it with them later or ask them to leave the public area with you to discuss it right away. If someone has kept you on hold for too long, ask that next time they take your number and call you back within 10 minutes. That way, you are not waiting on the line for them. If someone is talking down to you because they are more educated, quietly remind them that part of their role is to help you understand the vocabulary of their profession. Since they had to learn all those terms once themselves, it is now their turn to teach you.

When You Cannot Avoid Conflict

As conflict is inevitable and not necessarily negative, try the following steps to put the conflict in perspective.

- Remember that most conflicts are only a small part of your life and not worth the emotional energy we give to them.
- Do something to try to resolve the conflict even if it doesn't work. We use most of our emotional energy during conflicts on anger and frustration. Instead, use your creative energies to try to understand the other person's point of view and see how resolving the conflict can be **mutually** beneficial.
- Get away from the conflict to cool off. Try to place the conflict in perspective to the rest of your life and also in perspective to time. Will you remember this conflict next year? Will this conflict change your life in the next 10 years?
- Learn from the conflict. Whether the conflict is a win/lose situation or resolved to your mutual benefit, see if there are things you can learn from it to prevent or resolve similar

conflicts more quickly in the future.

- In extreme situations, evaluate whether or not your client may leave the situation.

Summary

- People always do the best they can with what they know at the time. Few, if any people wake up in the morning with the sole purpose of making your life miserable.
- The more we understand people the more we respect them even if we don't agree with them.
- The opposite of love is not hate but fear. So much behavior that we dislike is a result of our own fear or the fears of others.
- If you choose not to resolve conflicts, accept responsibility for your decision. This may include leaving the circumstances where the conflict occurs.
- When you resolve conflicts you do it for yourself and not for others.

- "Why do I always have to make the first move? It isn't fair!" Resolving conflicts has little to do with fairness. It has to do with seeing the opportunity and satisfaction of resolving conflicts for the benefit of your client and their family.

Your Notes on Mediation

Appendix 1. Questions to Ask

Questions Doctors Need Answered

You will probably see many doctors, nurses, pharmacists, and other caregivers during the length of an illness, medical condition, or recovery. They will all want some of the same answers to the following questions. If you have written them down in advance, it can save you time.

Some of these questions will work just as well in any system when properly adapted. **Make your own list for every appointment or telephone conversation or written communication you have with someone who can help you**.

- What concerns you about your condition today?

- What is the history of this

condition?

- Where in the body did the pain/ symptom begin?
- When did it start (date and time)?
- On a scale of 1-5, with 5 equaling the worst pain you have ever had (e.g., broken arm, appendicitis), how do you rate your pain?
- Describe any other symptoms you have had.
- What were you doing at the time of the pain/symptom?
- To what degree does your pain/ symptom limit your normal activities?
- How long does the pain/symptom last (an hour, all day)?
- Is the pain/symptom constant or does it change?
- Does the pain/symptom stay in one place or spread out to other parts of your body?
- What makes the pain/symptom worse?
- What makes the pain/symptom better?

- How do the following things affect your symptoms: bowel movements, urination, coughing, sneezing, breathing, swallowing, menstruation, exercise, walking, eating, sleeping, rest?
- What do you intuitively feel is wrong?
- Do you have any other information that might help me?
- Is there one thing we could do to make this situation bearable for you, until we sort through the whole dilemma?

Your Questions about Tests

Even though you are at home now, you may need to return to a hospital or clinic for further tests and treatments. The following questions will help you to understand your condition and have some control over what happens to you. That control will probably help you recover at home faster.

Studies have shown that people who are aware of the physical effects of a test or treatment are less afraid and recover more quickly from a difficult procedure than patients with little or no advance information. Although caregivers may not have had a particular test themselves, they can usually provide fairly detailed information based on other people's experiences and the medical literature available. It is important for a person to understand why a doctor has recommended a test and how the test is done. The following questions can be asked of a doctor, nurse, or technician to help the person decide whether or not to consent to the test.

- What is the purpose of this test?

- What do you expect to learn from this test? Will the results change my treatment in any way?
- What will the test feel like (any pain or discomfort)?

- What are the common risks involved in this test?
- Are there any aftereffects of this test?
- Can my spouse/child/friend come with me? If not, why not? (The medical world is slowly changing to allow someone to be with the patient during difficult tests. This change is similar to fathers now being permitted into delivery rooms.)
- Can I return home or to work after the test?
- When will I get the results of this test? Can I see you to go over them with you?
- What will happen to me if I choose not to take this test?
- What are the chances of error or false positive/negative results? (Some tests have a high incidence of "false positives." Often, tests cannot be definite but they can help doctors know if they are on the right track.)

- What are the costs involved, if any?
- Is there any preparation that I should be aware of before I go to the test?
- Are the facility and/or the machine used in the test accessible to me as: I use a wheelchair, I cannot see well, I am claustrophobic?
- Other questions.

Your Questions about Medications (Drugs)

You may ask your pharmacist or doctor the following questions. Some information is included with the medication. People are responsible for thinking about these questions whenever they are asked to take new drugs. Keep in mind that people react in different ways to medication.

Remember that not following the instructions carefully may lead to poor or even dangerous results.

Some of the answers to the following questions can be found in any of the standard pharmaceutical books listed in the reference section. If your pharmacist or doctor cannot answer your questions with enough detail, check one of the reference texts.

- What is the name and purpose of these drugs?
- What do the drugs actually do inside my body?
- Will the generic drug absorb in the same way as the name brand drug? If not, do I need a different dosage or different drug?
- Is there a less expensive generic version of these drugs?
- How often do I take the drugs each day and for how many days?
- What food, liquids, activities, and other drugs should I avoid when taking these drugs?
- What are the effects of mixing my various drugs together?

- What are the common and less common side-effects of these drugs?
- How can these side-effects be controlled?
- If this drug is a narcotic, should I also be getting a stool softener and/ or laxative, eating more fiber and drinking more liquids to prevent constipation?
- When should I return to give you feedback about the effectiveness of the drugs? How do I know when I should call you if the drugs produce side-effects?
- What will happen if I choose not to take these drugs?
- What are some non-pharmaceutical alternatives to taking drugs for my condition (e.g., herbal, body work, mind-body models)?
- What special storage instructions should I follow? (Pharmacists usually label medication with specific instructions but you should be sure that the labels are present.)
- Are there repeats on this

prescription? Can this prescription be repeated without coming to see you again?

- What are the costs involved? (Many prescriptions are never filled because people do not tell their doctors that they cannot afford the medication.)
- Do you know if my medical insurance covers any of these costs? (Ask your insurance agent or government insurance official this question.)
- What if my symptoms are relieved – should I keep taking my medications?
- What if I forget to take my medications? Do I double up or just skip a dose?
- What if I run out of medication? Who do I call for more – specialist, family doctor, or pharmacist?
- Other questions

Questions to Your Doctors about Your Condition

Once you have been physically examined and appropriate tests have been done, you will talk with your doctor about your condition. Having a family caregiver or advisor with you to take notes, ask questions, and advocate on your behalf is almost always recommended.

Your family doctor, as your advocate and mediator in the medical world, should help you understand the medical system. Why and how are tests done? What does the diagnosis of your condition mean to you? What treatment alternatives are there? What is the prognosis (prediction of the probable course of a disease) for your condition? What types of support (financial, physical, emotional, and spiritual) are available to you?

Try to get your family doctor actively

involved if you have trouble understanding or talking with your specialists. Always make sure that you understand what your doctors are saying. It is common for them to use terms you may not understand. Doctors had to learn what these terms meant when they went to school, so they can help you understand them too.

In order not to waste your doctor's time, it is important to ask specific questions. If you know your family doctor well, you might give him a copy of the following checklist of questions that you want answered, especially if your situation has changed dramatically since your last visit.

Fill in the answers to your questions (or get a family member or friend to do it for you) so you do not have to repeat the questions at a later point. Also ask for reference material that might answer some of the questions for you. This reduces the time commitment for your doctor and allows you to return later with even more specific questions and concerns. There are times, of course, when your doctor will be unable to give you specific answers because your disease may not be predictable. However, your doctor can offer some educated guesses with recommendations of where you can go to get further information.

Diagnosis

Diagnosis is not an exact science because there are too many unknown variables. This is why second opinions are sometimes necessary. Because health care depends on many people, a second or third set of eyes who have viewed the results of a test might lead to a diagnosis. Doctors can usually provide an accurate diagnosis with illnesses and conditions that have exacting scientific tests. One must be careful, however, that the tests were performed accurately and that the conclusions are confirmed before making major treatment decisions.

- What do I have?
- How did I get it?
- How can I prevent it from happening again or getting worse?

The Disease Itself

- Based on your experience and medical studies, what is the usual progress of this disease?
- What can I expect next?
- What other physical and mental abilities will be affected?
- Where can I learn more about this disease or condition?
- Can you recommend anyone I should see to get a second opinion?
- Other questions

Infections

- Can I give this illness to others? If so, how would they get it from me?

- Other questions

Other Possible Diseases

- Could the test results and symptoms indicate a different disease than the one we're discussing?
- Other questions

Treatment

- What treatment do you suggest?
- How does the treatment work?
- How will I evaluate its success or failure?
- How long after I begin the treatment should I see you again to report any progress?
- How often will I need the treatment?
- What are the side-effects of this treatment?
- What are some of the medical and non-medical alternatives to these treatments?

- What if I cannot afford this therapy or treatment? What are less expensive alternatives? How do the success rates compare? [Many therapies and treatments are covered by provincial and territorial health insurance. However, some treatments have more associated costs. For example, longer treatment in a hospital may require paying more parking fees which can be very expensive. Some treatments require "topping up" with a patient's own money if treatments go beyond what the insurance covers. For example, there are limited visits to chiropractors, registered massage therapists, and physiotherapists.)
- Other questions

Prognosis

Prognosis is a prediction of the probable course and outcome of a disease or condition. It is not an exact science. While you want to know what is probably going to happen to you, there are many variables that may give you a different outcome than what is expected in other people. Your body, mind, and spirit are unique and what happens to you may be very different than what happens to other people.

- What is the expected outcome of this illness?
- What will happen if I choose not to treat this illness through medication, surgery, or other treatments?
- What are the long-term effects of this illness?
- For shorter recovery periods, how long will it be before I can return to work and normal activities?
- Will I have pain as the disease develops?

- What is an educated guess as to how long I have to live?
- Other questions

Questions When You Go to a Hospital

When you go to a hospital, it is important to remember that you are there to receive a service. You remain in control of that service by consenting to, or refusing, the tests and treatments offered to you. You can refuse any and all treatments and tests offered, if you wish, unless you have a communicable disease that may harm others.

- If English is not my first language, is there anyone I can speak to in my own language to help me understand my medical care? [Family members are probably not the best translators but they can be good listeners to ensure person-centered care is happening and that translations are accurate.]

- What is the name of the admitting doctor who I can call if I need help? Who is the doctor in charge of my case and how can I reach them?
- Is the doctor in charge of my case a specialist, intern, resident, or medical student?
- What special rules and regulations should I be aware of while I am in this facility?
- What is the discharge procedure for leaving this facility? (You can leave whenever you decide but it may be against a hospital's wishes.)
- Is this a teaching hospital? If so, will anyone request that I participate in a research or educational program? (You have the right to consent or refuse to be part of any research or education program.)
- Does the hospital have a patient advocate office or social worker who can answer any of my questions about my hospital stay?

- What costs are involved in my hospital stay, if any?
- What are the visiting rules?
- Are the rooms clean?
- Will I get proper care for my other conditions?
- Will I be able to sleep at night in a quiet, dark room?
- Can I get food when I am hungry?
- Who else will be involved in my care (e.g., nurses, respiratory therapists, physiotherapists)?
- With whom can I discuss my care plan?
- With whom will you be discussing my care plan?
- Can a family member stay overnight with me?
- Other questions

Questions before Surgery

- Surgery is a frightening prospect for most people. If people understand the reasons for surgery, the procedures that are followed, and the results they can expect, then their fear and anxiety is greatly reduced. Studies have shown that people who understand what is happening to them recover more quickly and often feel less pain because of reduced anxiety. If you are having elective surgery, it is incredibly useful to speak to someone who has had it.

- What are the benefits and risks of this surgery?
- What are the alternatives, their benefits, and risks?
- What is the prognosis if I choose not to have surgery?
- Can you recommend a few people who have had this surgery who can help me prepare for it?
- What are the risks of anesthesia in my condition? When will the anesthesiologist meet with me to explain the procedures?
- What is the success rate for this surgery? What is the doctor's own

success rate with this surgery?

- What are the pre-surgery procedures?
- What happens during the actual surgery?
- What are the post-surgery procedures?
- Will I have much pain and discomfort after surgery?
- What things can I expect to see when I wake up, e.g., will I be on a ventilator, will I have blood transfusions, or will I be in the intensive care unit?
- What is the expected length of my recovery from surgery?
- How soon after surgery can I go to the bathroom, eat, walk, go home or to work, have sex, smoke, or drink alcohol?
- What are the names of the surgeons who will be operating?
- Will there be any medical students operating on me? (You have the option to refuse treatment by anyone other than your surgeon.

The benefit of having surgery in a teaching hospital is that you have highly skilled backup and overseers to the procedure that you may not have in a community hospital. The key is finding out how many similar procedures that surgeon has done or supervised.

- What are the costs involved, if any?
- What will happen after my hospital stay? Will I go to a rehabilitation center or go home and get homecare support? Who will coordinate this and will they be part of the planning early on to ensure continuity of care?
- Other questions

Appendix 2. Talking With Your Doctor and Other Health Professionals

Understanding the Doctor and Other Health Professionals

There is a natural apprehension by many people toward anything medical. In the past few years, however, there has been a heightened awareness that everyone benefits when the person and family work together with their professional caregivers. Open and honest communication relieves some anxiety for the person and their family, while the doctors and caregivers feel more job satisfaction and less personal stress.

Caregivers have stresses that everyone can help diminish by working together. The stresses of many professional caregivers include the following:

- heavy workload (it isn't enough to be a healthcare provider these days - you must also be a business person, a politician, and a bureaucrat)
- determining how much patients wish to know about their illness (although most people prefer to know the truth about their illness, there are those who prefer that the doctor not tell them the complete truth)
- the increasing administrative requirements of governments and insurance companies
- little time to learn new treatments and methods even though some professionals (e.g., doctors) must study a certain number of hours per year to keep their licenses
- little time for personal stress

reduction
- increasing numbers of lawsuits
- ambivalence or decreased public respect for medical/healthcare professionals in general

Some eminent doctors have written about doctor-patient relationships. Sir William Osler, 19th century Canadian doctor, diagnostician, and scholar believed that knowing what type of patient has a disease is more important than knowing what type of disease a patient has. He gave his patients little medication but lots of optimism.

Norman Cousins, in his book, *The Anatomy of an Illness,* described a visit he had with Dr. Albert Schweitzer in Africa. Schweitzer explained his philosophy of medical practice. He believed that people carry their own doctor inside of them. They go to see a doctor because they do not recognize their own strength. A physician's greatest asset is their ability to bring out the doctor within each patient. By helping patients gain a sense of personal control or mastery over their lives, doctors can also derive professional satisfaction that they are making a positive difference in the lives of their patients.

What Doctors Can Learn from You

There are many things doctors can learn from the person who is ill and from their families:

- **Facts about the person's condition.** This seems obvious, but some symptoms are not adequately addressed by the doctor because the person does not mention new symptoms, or is overly optimistic and feeling better for seeing the doctor. This may also be due to time constraints or assumptions that the doctor or the person makes about the condition.

- **New treatments.** You may have heard about new research that the doctor has not yet investigated. Sometimes these treatments are not proven but discussing them can get everyone more involved in treatment decisions. That sense of control can improve an ill person's self image and decrease their anxiety. Let the doctor know you wish to discuss the alternative options so they can book the appointment time appropriately.
- **Feedback on treatment**. People who are ill are always present for every symptom, test, treatment, and appointment over the months or years of treatment. They can offer vital feedback on their present treatments, feelings, and fears and must never be ignored.
- **Further treatment**. People who are ill must be encouraged by professional caregivers to express their needs and to help the caregivers determine further

treatment.

Some Dos and Don'ts of Improved Communication

From the perspectives of doctors and other professionals, there are proven techniques that people can use to improve the patient-care provider relationship. Some people will choose not to try the following suggestions and, in effect, choose not to communicate and cooperate.

Some Dos

- Know the care providers' names and help them remember yours.
- Communicate with the professionals about your physical, emotional, spiritual, and information needs.
- Cooperate fully once a decision on treatment is mutually decided.
- Write down the important questions to ask (usually in groups

of three to five to avoid overwhelming a care provider with too many questions). Record their answers or bring a loved one along and let them record the answers.

- Respect the caregiver's time while expecting the same in return.
- Ask specific questions rather than, "Why did this happen to me?"
- Offer a time limit for discussion (e.g., 7 minutes) and stick to it. In this way you build up a trusting relationship with the caregivers and they know you respect their time.

Some Don'ts

- Don't ignore medical instructions after a mutual decision has been made.
- Don't ask the same questions over and over again. It is better to record the professional's answers.
- Don't bring up questions about other family members and friends in hope of free medical advice.

- Don't keep telephoning one care provider with questions that can be better answered by another expert such as a nurse, pharmacist, or therapist.
- Don't wait until new pains or negative symptoms have become serious before communicating them.
- Don't forget to communicate emotional and spiritual needs rather than putting on a brave face.

- Don't see two doctors or specialists for the same condition. Choose a treatment option and stick with that doctor for consistent care.
- Don't follow other medical or alternative therapies without consulting the principal doctor, as different therapies may conflict. If your doctor disapproves and you still want to try alternative methods, get another doctor who is more comfortable working in this way.

- Don't forget to treat the care providers with respect and concern.

The Differences between Family Physicians and Specialists

- Your *family physician* is responsible for your initial care and diagnosis and for follow-up after treatment by specialists. Some are able to go to the hospital and speak on your behalf with their colleagues and others are not, depending on the rules within your healthcare community.
- Your *specialist(s)* are responsible for the diagnosis and treatment of specific illnesses or conditions. When you have more than one condition or illness, you will have several specialists who may, or may not, talk to each other about your care.

- Specialists plan your treatment and family physicians help explain and monitor treatment and send you back to specialist(s) for further care, if necessary.
- For both types of physicians you will have initial appointments of about 15-30 minutes and then follow-up appointments of about 5-6 minutes. This time is valuable so use it well. You will need to write out your questions and concerns and have a family member or friend come with you to write down the answers during the appointment.

Some Tips When Dealing With Specialists

Bring a summary of your medical history with you to each appointment, especially noting what has happened in the last year. Keep an ongoing log so you can send a copy to the doctor or community agency, and add to it as things change.

Bring your medications with you to every appointment so the doctor can verify the drug and dosage and see what other physicians have prescribed since you last met.

Ask your specialist for either written material or references where you can get more answers to your concerns and questions. For example, if you have recently been diagnosed with diabetes, your specialist cannot explain everything about the condition in a short appointment. However, they can provide you with written material, perhaps even a video or audiotape with common information you will need to know, or refer you to a specific patient information clinic. Once you know more about your condition, you can discuss specific concerns not answered in the general information.

It may be hard to reach your specialist when you are in the middle of treatment. Here are some tips:

- If you are in hospital, ask the nurse

in charge to contact your specialist for you or ask to speak to the physician whose name is on your wristband (who is responsible for coordinating your care while you are in the hospital). You may also ask the charge nurse or specialist when they are usually at the hospital so that you can contact them at that time rather than when they have office hours.

- If you are at home, ask the nurse/receptionist in the office to have the specialist call you. Many specialists do not mind talking to you once a day during a particularly difficult time for you, but more than that is too difficult for them to manage. You should only call them when they are the only person who can help (versus talking with a nurse, homecare case manager, social worker, pharmacist, physiotherapist).
- Have one family member act as the family's spokesperson (perhaps

with a backup liaison for times when this person is not available) so that the physician does not have to give the same answers to multiple people. Ideally, this person will be flexible enough to be at the hospital when the physician has rounds and will have some understanding of health care.

- Arrange for a family meeting with the specialist (or specialists if more are involved in the care), responsible nurses, and other professionals to deal with unanswered concerns and questions. The hospital social worker may coordinate such a meeting.
- If you have concerns, write them out for the charge nurse or office nurse/receptionist so that the physician can prioritize their calls. You can imagine that many people want to speak with the specialist so they have to decide who gets called first. They often make their calls at

the end of their office hours. Also leave them the times of day when you are easiest to reach and the telephone number.

- Some physicians will give out their e-mail address so questions can be answered by e-mail. This is particularly helpful for factual questions like "When should I be taking these various drugs during the day and do I take them with food or not?"
- It is not helpful to show up to an appointment with a large pile of research you have done at the library or on the internet. If you are going to the internet for information, choose reliable sites like those at the back of this book. Narrow down your questions and ideas to reasonably fit into the time you have. Many physicians subscribe to their own internet sources for up-to-date medical information. Ask them to print off relevant sections for you.

- Your specialist does not control the resources of the hospital so their operating room time and the tests that need to be done are not always under their control. The more senior the physician, the more control they have over scheduling. However, emergencies and unexpected equipment delays or repairs play a large part in who gets what treatment or test and when.
- If your concerns are urgent or you have had difficulty getting in touch with your physician, become more assertive and make reasonable demands with deadlines so that the physician understands your urgency. If you cannot be assertive yourself, then ask your family spokesperson to do so. It is a universal truth that people often respond to patients with the greatest need or the loudest demands (the squeaky wheel gets the grease). If you are reasonable and assertive, you will have a better

chance of having your concerns and needs met. There is also some benefit in being kind to others. If you want to be treated well, treat your professional caregivers well.

Resolving Communication Problems

When open communication does not seem possible, there are other options available. If the problem has become serious, bring in the community or hospital social worker, the hospital discharge planner, or the homecare case manager to see if improvements can be made.

Other caregivers, such as a cleric, nurse, occupational therapist, case manager, or patient advocate may also be helpful. They may call a "case conference" so that everyone involved can work through any difficulties. [See the Mediation section in the *navCare*

Textbook.]

When the communication cannot be improved, the person and family can do one or more of the following (although during such an emotional time these suggestions will not be easy to follow):

- Change specialists or doctors on the advice of another caregiver. Keep your existing specialist until you have found another one so that care continues.
- Change hospitals or the service you are using.
- If there are no alternatives available where you live, ask a family member or friend to become an assertive advocate on your behalf to speak to the caregiver, patient representative, ombudsperson, or the organization's president or executive director. The advocate must not stop until they are successful.
- If it is the person or family that is

uncooperative, the doctor might recommend a different doctor or hospital. They must legally continue care until the patient has found a new doctor.

- Many communication problems are not the fault of just one person. People have different personalities and for whatever reason, some people do not communicate well with each other. In the case of family members, a doctor may find it easier to speak to a single member of the family than to the whole family at once. Recognizing that the person is the doctor's most important concern, the family can arrange to choose a member to act as spokesperson and minimize the time a doctor needs to spend with the whole family.

After all the studies have been read, the personal experiences related, and the advice given, the underlying principle of total care of the person who is ill or recovering remains cooperation between patient, family, and caregivers. A mutual respect and understanding of each other's feelings and needs will result in a fuller life for the person who is ill and personal satisfaction for the family members and caregivers that they have helped the patient to the best of their abilities.

Your Notes on Talking with Professionals

Appendix 3. Powers of Attorney

Different provinces, territories, and countries have different regulations about how someone can legally delegate someone else to speak for them if they ever become legally unable to speak for themselves. For example, if you are in an accident and can't speak, you can have a legal document that says that your spouse, parent, or best friend can make decisions on your behalf.

The following information is accurate for Ontario. Your lawyer can write up the form or you can use the Ministry of the Attorney General's standard form available through its booklet:

Office of the Public Guardian and Trustee. (2012) *Powers of Attorney."* Queen's Printer for Ontario. 21-page document at:

http://
www.attorneygeneral.jus.gov.on.ca/
english/family/pgt/poa.pdf

The Ministry also has a helpful brief "Question and Answer" guide to answer the most common questions at:

http://
www.attorneygeneral.jus.gov.on.ca/
english/family/pgt/livingwillqa.pdf

To learn more about the Substitute Decisions Act: http://
www.attorneygeneral.jus.gov.on.ca/
english/family/pgt/pgtsda.pdf

Encourage anyone who agrees to act as your power of attorney or substitute decision maker to go to these websites to download the same materials to learn what responsibilities they are agreeing to take on.

Do not use kits sold in stores as they may not have the legal wording required in your province or territory.

Powers of Attorney give written

directions about what a person may want in different situations. As legal tools they leave many unanswered questions. As communication tools, they encourage people to talk about what they want and still leave enough room for flexibility as situations change.

A Power of Attorney document gives a designated family member or another trusted person the right to make legal decisions in situations where the person cannot decide for themselves.

There are generally two types of Power of Attorney documents: Power of Attorney for Personal Care and Power of Attorney for Property. The first deals with **personal care** concerns including healthcare decisions (treatment and services), homecare decisions, food, living arrangements, housing, clothing, hygiene, safety, and life and death decisions. The Power of Attorney for Property deals with **financial, banking, insurance, and**

other legal issues.

The **Power of Attorney for Property** takes effect immediately upon signing unless you specify otherwise (e.g., only when you become legally incompetent to make financial and legal decisions yourself). The **Power of Attorney for Personal Care** comes into effect when you cannot make decisions any more (e.g., when you are in a coma or are legally declared incompetent) and stops when you are capable of making decisions for yourself again (e.g., after you recover from a coma).

Note that some institutions (e.g., banks and long-term care facilities) may try to have you sign their Power of Attorney for Property form including a clause the revokes any existing forms you have already signed. Rather than do that, offer to give them a copy of the Power of Attorney form you have already signed to add to your file.

It is also often suggested that one person should not have authority over both these general categories, as there may be a conflict of interest. For example, one might be less likely to demand certain medical interventions if they know it will deplete a person's financial savings. By splitting up the two categories, there are at least two people who can speak up for the person who is ill. This may not always be practical when the person has only a spouse, child, or friend to act in both capacities. It is especially important in this circumstance to have honest and open communication about what the person does, and does not, want done in various situations. In cases of dispute, the law generally recognizes the Power of Attorney for Personal Care over the Power of Attorney for Property.

The person you designate is often referred to legally as a **substitute decision maker**. There are rules about who cannot act as your substitute decision maker and who cannot witness your Power of Attorney. Ask your lawyer for advice or use the forms approved by your province and state that lists who can, and who cannot, act for you. These are available from bookstores, government offices, libraries, software packages, or through your lawyer.

If you travel a lot and are likely to be outside your home province or state, you should get a lawyer to look into whether your Powers of Attorney will be valid in the places you intend to visit.

Each province and state has different rules in place about Powers of Attorney. You can make up your own form but be sure that you follow your local governmental regulations about the correct format and language of these legal documents to minimize errors. Even a signature in the wrong place can negate these forms. Get a legal form from bookstores, government offices or website, libraries, software packages, or through your lawyer.

Power of Attorney documents name the person who will make substitute decisions for you. There are also documents called **Living Wills**. These documents state in writing what you want done in certain medical emergencies (e.g., whether you want to receive blood transfusions, be resuscitated if you stop breathing, put on life support systems temporarily). They **are not** legally binding documents but do express to your substitute decision maker what you would like to happen in certain situations.

Everyone should have these Powers of Attorney. These legal documents provide the hospital, financial systems, and the courts with a person who can make decisions on behalf of the patient should the patient be unconscious, incapable of communication, or mentally incompetent to make decisions.

Here are some things to consider:

- The person signing these forms may want to set a time limit on some of their specific instructions. For example, if they instruct their attorney to allow the healthcare team to try any and all treatment options to keep them alive, they may add the time limit of three months (or any time period). If, after that time, they are still unable to speak for themselves and their power of attorney and the medical care team all agree that any further treatment is hopeless, they give their attorney the authority to stop all (or some — depending on the person) treatments and life-sustaining efforts. For many people, this will prevent having life support treatments go on for months or years.
- These documents may include the

instruction that if the person is found dead after a heart attack, with no one present when they died, that they request that no one performs CPR.

- They may also include that the person wants, or does not want, a Do Not Resuscitate order in their medical file to be changed only with the consent of their power of attorney (i.e., no unilateral decision by healthcare providers).
- If appointing more than one attorney, the person can decide whether the attorneys must agree on all decisions or whether either can decide for them. They may choose the second option if, for example, their two children travel a lot and only one is likely to be nearby to make decisions on their behalf.
- What happens if your loved one does not have a signed Power of Attorney? There is a typical priority order that the courts use to

determine who gets to decide. In Ontario, the law is called the Substitute Decisions Act. Each province and territory has their own rules. Typically the order is:

1. Power of attorney
2. Spouse (living together in a married or common-law relationship)
3. Parent or child(ren) – equally powerful
4. Siblings
5. Other relatives.

If there is conflict within the family, hospital staff may bring in a social worker or mediator to help solve the conflict regarding decision-making.

For more information about advance care planning, please go to your provincial / territorial Attorney General's website, the Advocacy Centre for the Elderly (www.advocacycentreelderly.org or the Canadian Hospice Palliative Care Association: www.advancecareplanning.ca.

Appendix 4. Basic Healthcare Navigation: Going to the Emergency Department

There are two ways to get to a hospital emergency department for an assessment (although this does not guarantee the patient will be admitted):

1. By ambulance (either by calling 911 or by calling an ambulance directly for non-emergency transfers)
2. By being driven, or driving yourself, to the hospital Emergency Department

Pros and Cons of Both

Ambulance drivers may not take you to the hospital of your choice and your family will be forced to follow you. The ambulance may be redirected to a different hospital. On the other hand, the paramedics may know the city hospital with the best reputation for dealing with, for instance, cardiac patients. People arriving by ambulance tend to get placed in a hospital bed faster than patients who drive themselves in because the ambulance needs their gurney back.

Driving yourself (or being driven by a family member or friend) allows you to go right away and go to the hospital of your choice. The disadvantage is that you may not know which hospital is best and the wait time could be longer.

What to bring with you:

- MOST IMPORTANT: someone to take notes, answer questions if you cannot speak for yourself, and advocate for you

- all of your medications in a bag
- any notes you have on your medical history
- the names of your family doctor and specialists
- money for parking (it seems silly but many people get stuck without enough money to pay to leave the hospital parking lot)
- a cell phone with important numbers uploaded so you don't need to remember them. Hospitals may ask you to not to use them, or to step away from certain areas before using them, but there are no studies that indicate that cell phones interrupt medical equipment. Use them sparingly and quietly.

What happens when you get to the Emergency Department?

Typically, you will first see a triage nurse. This person has to determine who gets seen first based on how sick they are. Someone with a cut hand will have to wait until the person with a heart problem has been seen. It is NOT on a first-come, first-served basis. That's only fair.

However, many patients will not give enough information to the triage nurse, so she or he cannot make a good judgment. If you have chest pains, had a recent fall, or are short of breath, you must be seen right away. You may think you can wait, but you probably cannot. When the triage nurse asks, "How are you?", answer with complete truthfulness in order for the nurse to make a complete and accurate assessment of your condition. This is not the time to be shy or proud – you are there for help, so get it as quickly as possible.

Once you are called from the waiting area (assuming you had to wait), you will go into the actual department. You will likely be in a large ward with curtained-off areas for each patient or into a separate small room. You can wait there for quite some time as well. If you wait for more than 15 minutes, ask the person who has come with you to go to the nurses' station and ask when you might be seen and whether you can have something to eat or drink (not likely, but it will tell them you've been waiting a while and are thirsty).

If the room is chilly (it often is), ask for a warm blanket. They have a special machine for that, and it also gets them to think about you. You might ask for an extra pillow for neck or back support if that would help.

Either an Emergency Specialist doctor, who works full-time in the hospital, will see you or you may get a Family Physician doing their monthly shift rotation in the Emergency Department. Either can help you although the specialist may be most involved in very serious trauma cases.

Your family member or friend as advocate

This person can help distract you, if you have to wait a long time. Also, they can be comforting and supportive and ask for help should they determine you need it faster.

They need to be calm but persistent. They are not there to make friends but they can be friendly. If they raise their voice in frustration, they must do it in a controlled way. Uncontrolled aggression or anger will not get the same results as controlled, assertive communication.

Test

Likely some tests will need to be done for a starting diagnosis that may take some time. Ask that your family member or friend stays with you to keep you company and provide assistance if needed.

After diagnosis

Once the doctor has a starting diagnosis they will either tell you what it is and send you home with further instruction (typically, "See your family doctor as soon as you can") or admit you to the hospital. If they admit you, you will be transferred to a specific floor or ward where staff will care for your specific needs. If a bed is not available, you may have to spend a day or two in the emergency department.

If you are admitted you will likely never see the emergency doctor again. Many hospitals now have "hospitalists" who are Family Doctors who have decided to work 9-5 in a hospital rather than run their own practices. They may be responsible for your overall care while in hospital. Specialists are responsible for their specific area of expertise.

The more complex your case, the more doctors will be involved in your care.

You and your family members or friends who are supporting you will be the only people with the "whole" picture of personal need. Many specialists, for example, may not read what other doctors have written in your medical file. Each has their own piece of the puzzle before them. That's why you might have to answer the same questions over and over again.

It will be a major healthcare improvement when one doctor is assigned to oversee all of your care from start to finish in the hospital using an electronic file to keep everyone up to date, including the patient and their family caregivers. Not all hospitals do that yet so it is important to know as much as possible about the care being provided.

Pain Control

The key thing for you to know about pain control is that no one needs to suffer unbearable pain. You may have to have some pain as you go through tests and such (i.e., they cannot give you pain medication until they know what is causing the pain – the pain helps them determine what is wrong).

But once you are diagnosed, ask for sufficient pain medication so that your pain is well controlled. If you cannot move because of pain or are constantly moaning or yelling from the pain, it is obviously not well controlled. This is when having a family member or advisor with you to advocate on your behalf is particularly helpful.

When Problems Arise

There are several people who can help you when a problem arises. The more you remember people's names and help them remember yours, the better your care with be.

No matter how wonderful people are in providing your care, there will be errors and there will be conflicts. So start with your nurse and ask her or him for specific help. If they cannot be helpful enough, there are some other things you can try:

- In the emergency departments of some hospitals there are now GEM nurses: Geriatric Emergency Managers. This applies only for older patients but at least that population now has someone specific who can be helpful and advocate on their behalf.
- Talk to the doctor with whom you have most contact. If you are having difficulties or are in an emergency, do not be afraid to ask the closest medical professional for help.
- Social workers have professional relationships with other staff members (e.g., doctors, nurses, physiotherapists, and occupational therapists) and can help mediate conflicts within the hospital.
- Some of the most helpful and knowledgeable people in a hospital are the porters, clinical clerks

(secretaries), cleaning staff, meal servers, and volunteers. They understand the power structures on a floor and know who can get what you need fastest.

- The Head Nurse (this person has different titles in different hospitals) has responsibility for the nursing care in a hospital unit and would be a good person to approach regarding any concerns about your nursing care.
- The Director of Nursing oversees all aspects of nursing in the hospital. If you have spoken with the head/ charge nurse and your issue has still not been resolved, the director of nursing would be your next best problem solver.
- Some hospitals have "patient advocates" or "patient representatives." They can do some things for you that others cannot.
- Chaplains can be a wealth of information and support whether they represent your specific faith or

not. They can be advocates without having the same faith as you.

Your family doctor, whether or not they can visit you in the hospital, can make a few phone calls to get you answers to your questions. Sometimes it just takes a doctor talking with another doctor to get the information needed.

Only in extreme cases do you bring in a lawyer or mediator to represent your concerns. People don't like the threat of being sued, nor do they like controversy. If your requests are reasonable and not threatening, then a lawyer's presence can speed things along. Most institutions would rather smooth over difficulties than drag them through the legal system. That said, hospitals use large law firms and have what seems like unlimited budgets to fight a patient's lawyer. You want a lawyer working for you who understands that and who has experience negotiating in good faith for a quick and practical solution to your needs.

Minimizing Conflicts

People in health care can be overworked, feel undervalued and, just like the rest of us, really appreciate the common courtesies of "thank you," "please," and "I'm sorry." They appreciate a genuine offer of flowers, healthy (and not-so-healthy) foods, and something that says, "We appreciate what you are doing for us." This is just the same for everyone else in our world. However, in health care the demands and needs are high and the professionals do not often feel truly appreciated. You can help them with that, not just to get better care but also to improve the overall working and healing environment for everyone.

Your Notes on Basic Health Navigation

Appendix 5. Finding Out About Local Home and Healthcare Programs

Home care is a group of services to help people live at home when they are ill or recovering from an illness or surgery rather than staying in a hospital or long-term care facility.

Basic Services

- Visiting Nurses
- Personal Care Support Workers
- Home Support (help with homemaking such as light housekeeping, shopping, cooking, laundry)
- Physiotherapy
- Occupational Therapy
- Respiratory Therapy
- Social Work Counseling
- Speech Language Therapy
- Nutritional Counseling
- Housing Registry
- Personal Emergency Response Systems

Complex Services

- Home Intravenous Antibiotic Therapy
- Life Support/Ventilator Assistance Systems
- Services for Children with Complex Needs
- Tube Feedings (either by nose or through the stomach wall)
- Home Cancer Therapy
  Palliative Hospice Care or End-of-life Care
- Care for People with Dementia

Community Support Services

- Adult Day Centers
- Meals-on-Wheels and/or Wheels to Meals Programs
- Respite Care (so that caregivers can have some time off)
- Transportation help
  Help with shopping
  Help with home maintenance
- Volunteers

Homecare programs across Canada and the United States provide different services. To find out what is available in your community, you can check with your family doctor, local health authority, or other home healthcare providers. If a particular service is not available in your community, ask your political leaders why and how your community can arrange to get such service in the near future.

Communication Notes

Whenever you talk by telephone, in writing, or in person, keep a record of the conversation. You can use the following form as a guideline.

[Photocopy as many as you need.]

Date & Time ______________________________

Their name________________________________

Job Title __________________________________

Organization ______________________________

Items discussed:

Decisions and / or plans agreed to:

Resources

Telephone Helplines

To get healthcare information personally by telephone rather than looking at books or the internet, try the following:

Telehealth in Ontario: **1.866.797.0000** A nurse will answer your questions and advise you on whether you need to go to an Emergency Department right away, see your doctor within 24-48 hours, go to a walk-in medical clinic, or rest at home and call them back within 24-48 hours.

Call **211** for information on health & community services in your area and a representative will help you locate services nearby. You can also go to their website: www.211.ca .

Ask Elizabeth: **1.855.275.3549** is a service of the Saint Elizabeth Health Information charity. A nurse will answer more general questions on all health related matters.

For **homecare** services through your local CCAC (in Ontario) dial 310.2222 (no area code).

Written and Multimedia Resources

Top Books to Have Handy

Whenever looking at healthcare information, beware that some of the information that you will read may be disturbing. Always check with a doctor to make sure that the information you have researched on your own is accurate for **your particular situation**. You are not a statistic. There are many variables that define how someone might deal with an illness, condition, or disease.

Conlon, Patrick. (2009). *The essential hospital handbook: How to be an effective partner in a loved one's care.* New Haven: Yale University Press. [Canadian book]

Mayo Clinic family health book. (get latest ed.). New York: William Morrow. Extensive illustrated home medical reference including diagnosis, prevention, treatment alternatives, and more.

van Bommel, Harry. (2006). *Caring for loved ones at home: An illustrated, easy-to-follow guide to short and long-term care.* Toronto: Legacies Inc. Basic home nursing guide for family caregivers.

van Bommel, Harry. (2006). *Family hospice care: Pre-planning and care guide.* Toronto: Legacies Inc. Comprehensive guide for family caregivers to pre-plan with their loved one how they want to live until they die including meeting their physical, emotional, spiritual, and information needs.

NOTE: van Bommel's healthcare books, plus a dozen more, are available for FREE reading online at: www.carelibrary.com.

The Internet

A note of caution: Thousands of websites offer healthcare information. The information on some sites may not be accurate or current. Check to see who produces the website, their qualifications, and their credibility before assuming the information is correct. Like a journalist, always look for three trusted sources before accepting something as fact.

Health Information Sites

Canadian Healthcare Network
www.**canadianhealthcarenetwork**.ca
A general health information site with links to many other health-related sites.

Canadian Mental Health Association (CMHA)
www.cmha.ca
Authoritative site on mental health concerns.

Drugs.com

www.drugs.com

Senior editorial board members are pharmacists in Australia and New Zealand but their goal is to be the internet's most trusted resource for independent, objective, comprehensive, and up-to-date drug and related health information for both consumers and healthcare professionals. ***Verify facts with your own pharmacists.***

Health Canada's Information Site

www.hc-sc.gc.ca

The Canadian government's official site with many links to other reputable sites.

Mayo Clinic.Com

www.mayoclinic.com

An outstanding site for general health information. Often referenced by successful navigators/advisors and healthcare professionals.

Consumer Organizations

The Family Caregiver http://www.thefamilycaregiver.com
Canada's homecare and family caregiving resource center including resource guides on *Going Home* from the hospital and *The Home and Vehicle Modification Guide*. The are also archives of past magazine issues.

Patients Canada http://www.patientscanada.ca

Canada's national patient-led consumer organization to help patients impact and change healthcare systems for the better.

Saint Elizabeth www.saintelizabeth.com, and http://www.saintelizabeth.com/Health-Info/Ask-Elizabeth.aspx

A leader in providing caregiver support information through the Caregiver Compass, Caring for Family website and *Ask Elizabeth,* a caregiver support and information service to ask questions about health and community services in Ontario. 1.855.Ask Eliz (275-3549) or chat online at www.saintelizabeth.com.

Social Assistance

Check Blue government pages of your telephone book. Also:

www.211.ca a database of community, social, and health services.
Also Healthline at:
www.thehealthline.ca which puts health and community services at your fingertips for people of Ontario.

Legal Websites

e-Laws provides access to official copies of Ontario's statutes and regulations.

www.e-laws.gov.on.ca

Your Favorite Websites/ Resources

Acknowledgements

Our special gratitude to **Louise LeBlanc**, *navCare*'s project coordinator for pulling all of us together to produce something quite unique.

Thanks to **Dr. Michele Chaban**, **Janice Waugh** and **Tracey Nesbitt** for their thorough edits of all of the *navCare* materials as well as their original help in conceptualizing the work. Thanks to **Simon Constam** for proofreading the design version.

Thanks also to all of our ***navCare*** **partners** for contributing so freely of their time and content resources so that this truly is a collaborative project.

One of the key benefits of researching and writing this *navCare Series* is that one gets an opportunity to interview incredibly resourceful and creative people who freely share their information in the hopes of helping others. We are sincerely grateful to all the people who helped us through interviews, email exchanges, our survey and/or through reviewing drafts of our materials.

211 Ontario by Findhelp Information Services: **Faed Hendry**, Manager of Training and Outreach.

311 Toronto: **Heather Callahan**, Manager of Business Applications & Performance Accountability; City of Toronto; **Esther Noboa**, Supervisor; and **Tracy Smith**, Business Analyst.

ALS Society of Canada: **Oana Istoc**, Client Services Coordinator.

Better Living Health and Community Services: **Dena Silverberg,** Vice-President, Hospice and Social Services; **Sheila Berry**, Case Manager.

Caregiver Omnimedia Incorporated: **Don Fenn**, President and **Terry Morgan**, Executive Vice-President of Strategic Relationships, **Annie Fenn**, and **Stuart Teather**.

Michele Chaban, MSW, PhD is one of Canada's leading psychosocial experts in hospice palliative care and a leading mentor and teacher of mindfulness meditation in academic and healthcare settings (i.e., University of Toronto and McMaster University in Hamilton, Ontario, and Mount Sinai Hospital in Toronto).

Community Care Durham: **Cheryl MacLeod**, Manager, Planning and Partnerships.

Father William Cruse, a retired Anglican priest and family caregiver.

Deohaeko Support Network: **Janet Klees**, Family Coordinator.

Durham Association of Family Respite Services: **Peter Dill**, former Executive Director; **Teresa Dale**, Manager of Family Supports; **Cathy Bloomfield**, Family Support Facilitator.

Durham Family Network: **Helen Dionne**, Coordinator; **Tracy MacGillivray** (parent and advocate), **Eleanor Werner** (parent and advocate).

Julie M. Foley, former Executive Director of the Scarborough CCAC and Interim Executive Director of Ewart Angus Homes.

Dr. Gillian Gilchrist, former medical director of the palliative care service at Oshawa General Hospital.

Heart and Stroke Foundation of Ontario: **Beverly Powell-Vinden**, Manager, Mission Information.

Maureen Hennessy, of Hennessy Consulting and former senior executive at several healthcare facilities.

Hospice Toronto: **Dena Maule**, Executive Director; **Belinda Marchese,** Director of Clinical Services; **Sally Blainey**, Manager of Volunteer Services; and **Joyce Edem**, Coordinator of the Creating Caring Communities Program.

Diane Huson, family caregiver and client.

Metropolitan United Church: **Rev. Dr. John Joseph Mastandrea,** minister of spiritual growth and pastoral care development.

Novus Health: **Mira Jelic**, Co-Founder and Vice-President, Client Services.

Ontario Ministry of the Attorney General, Provincial Family Court: eight professionals representing crown attorneys, duty councils, and youth workers.

Parkinson Society Central & Northern Ontario: **Louise LeBlanc**, Volunteer Coordinator; **Robert TerSteege**, Informational and Referral Associate; clients: **Keith Goobie, Alice Betty Rustin, John Paul Scott**; and family care partner

Roslyn Patrick.

Patients Canada: **Rosalee Berlin**, Nursing Consultant and Educator and founder of *The Non-Smokers Rights Association* in Canada; **Jennifer Carroll**, Project Coordinator; **Brian Clark**, Patient Advocate; **Sholom Glouberman**, President; **Emily Nicholas**, Patient Advocate; and **Christina Spencer**, Communications Coordinator.

Dr. Laura Rotman, family physician.

Saint Elizabeth Health Care: **Nicole Beben**, VP, Knowledge & Care; **Pat Malone**, Integrity Officer; **Karen Ray**, Manager, Knowledge Translation; **Natalie Strouth**, Coordinator of the *Ask Elizabeth* project.

John and Toni Scully. John Scully is the author of *Am I Sane Yet?* – a book looking at mental health services. Toni is John's wife and a family care partner.

Sunnybrook Health Sciences Centre: **Lisa Priest**, Manager, Community Engagement & Patient Navigation, former journalist and author of *Operating in the Dark*.

Sykes Assistance Services Corporation: **Adam Jones**, Director of Client Relations and Privacy Officer; **Chantal Szydlik**, Community Resource Database Coordinator, internal database of community healthcare organization information that nurses use in helping callers and **Melissa Masson**, Clinical Practice Manager oversees call process, educator, operational manager and front line nurse in *Telehealth*.

Our sincere thanks to everyone who contributed their thoughts and ideas to our survey of clients and family caregivers. One of the keys to successful navigation is following the tried and tested paths of people who navigated similar journeys before you. That they share their stories so freely, is a gift to all of us.

Index

For further information on any aspect of the *navCare* 7-Volume Series, please contact us at

One at a Time Press:

oneatatimepress@dafrs.com

or visit our website:

www.dafrs.com

Made in the USA
Monee, IL
04 November 2026

67386412R00134